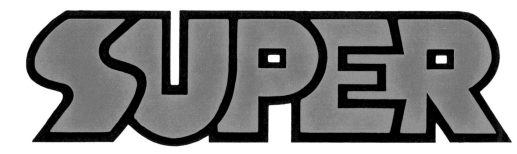

SUPERHEALTH
A challenge for all the family

JOHNSTON & BACON

LONDON & EDINBURGH

In association with Mazola Information Bureau

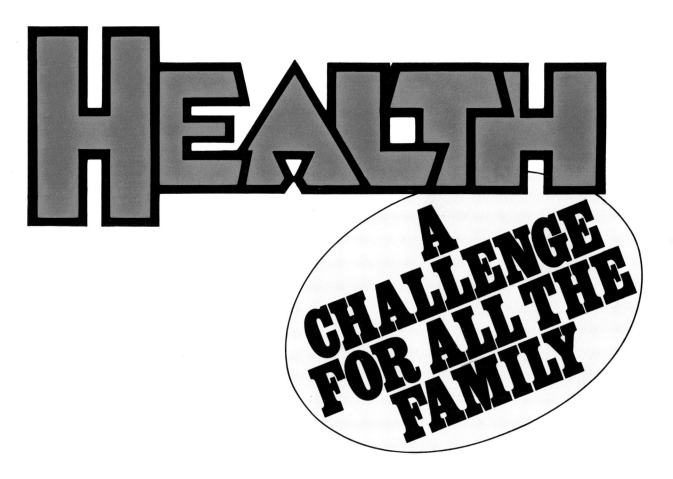

HEALTH
A CHALLENGE FOR ALL THE FAMILY

William and Janet Horwood

A Johnston and Bacon book published by
Cassell Ltd
35 Red Lion Square,
London WC1R 4SG
and
Tanfield House,
Tanfield Lane,
Edinburgh EH3 5LL
and at
Sydney, Auckland, Toronto, Johannesburg,
an affiliate of
Macmillan Publishing Co Inc,
New York

Text © William and Janet Horwood 1979
Design and illustrations © Diagram Visual
Information Ltd 1979
Art Director Kathleen McDougall

Typeset by
SX Composing Ltd
Rayleigh, Essex
Printed and bound in Great Britain by
Cambridge University Press,
Cambridge.

ISBN: 0 7179 4257 0
First published 1979

CONTENTS

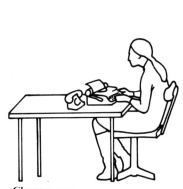

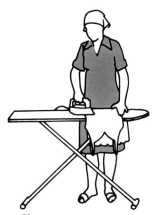

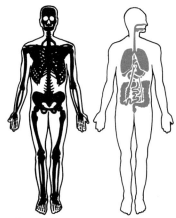

Note: This book is not intended as a substitute for the medical advice of physicians. The reader should regularly consult a physician in matters relating to health, particularly if unusual symptoms develop.

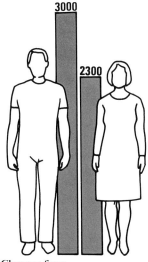

Chapter four
FOOD FOR HEALTH

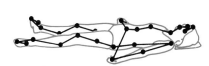

Chapter five
ROUTINES FOR RELAXATION

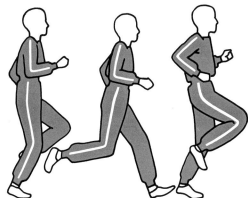

Chapter six
SUCCESSFUL EXERCISE

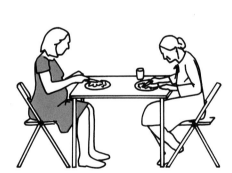

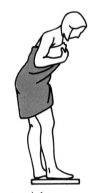

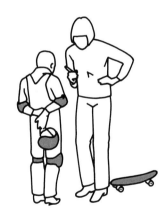

INTRODUCTION

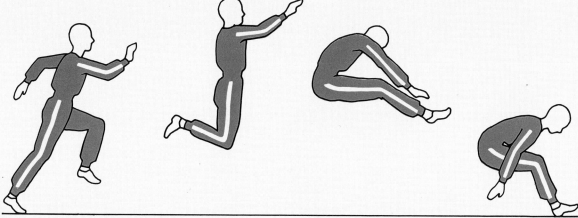

Superhealth is the ability to enjoy life to the full with a healthy mind and body which are in tune with each other. It's a rare quality which too few people possess, and one which many have never even witnessed in others they know. For we live in an unhealthy society where our lifestyles, the food we eat and the conditions we tolerate make it very hard to be fully healthy. The queues in doctors' surgeries, the millions of pounds spent on self-medication, and statistics on illness and disease all show how far from wholehealth most people are. What's worse is the fact that many of us seem prepared passively to accept a degree of ill-health all our lives **and not do much about it**. We have 'always had a pain in the lower back' or we 'always get two or three colds in the winter' or we 'couldn't get to sleep without these pills'. Few of us ask ourselves whether we might be much more healthy than we are. And of those that do probably a majority find the challenge of winning health in a polluted and stressed environment too great. We prefer to stay with the habits and lifestyle that allow us to do little more than muddle through life from a health point of view, rather than really to try to change things for ourselves. We know we are unfit, but we have too little will to do anything about it; we know we are over-

weight, but dieting is too hard. But, happily, things are changing. More and more people, especially in younger age groups, are now unwilling to accept second best from their bodies, or minds. Greater leisure time and a growing awareness of individual health needs are making people sit up and think . . . and wonder what steps can be taken towards wholehealth. This book is for them; for those of us who want to take a positive attitude about health. None of us – or very few – expect to be Olympic athletes, or to live a life completely free from illness or the occasional ache and pain. But we can expect to live a far more fulfilling life if we take the health challenge seriously and not as just another fad to talk about for a week or two and then forget. We believe that whatever your age, sex or circumstances you can benefit from the exciting process of asking questions about the basic things that affect your health – your food, your exercise and your lifestyle. This book helps you do this by raising the questions and showing you some of the answers. It is a guidebook rather than a do-it-yourself manual; a series of ideas rather than a dogmatic treatise. Most of all, it is an invitation to start on a journey towards wholehealth which, though it may sometimes be hard work, will never be boring.

ASK YOURSELF A FEW QUESTIONS

If you can answer 'yes' to all the following questions then you are physically and mentally healthy. If you **can't** answer them all positively don't worry, it means you are in the same boat as the majority of people; and, as this book shows, there is plenty you can do about it. But a word of warning: this is not a competitive quiz in which you are trying to do better than someone else; it's designed to help you start answering the simple question which most people who think about their general health ask at some time: 'Am I as healthy as I could be?' As the questions suggest, whole-health is a combination of physical and mental health. Because physical fitness is the easiest aspect of health to measure (and in some ways the easiest to do something about) we tend to measure our health as a whole in terms of our physical fitness. In practice, many of our physical ills are a reflection of the mental stress we live under so that a régime of keep-fit exercises may not prove the magic cure for our general state of health we hope it will be. You should not strain to answer each of the questions with a 'yes'. If the physical ones don't come easily and naturally, and there is any doubt in your mind about the answers to the others, then mark a firm 'no' on your scoresheet

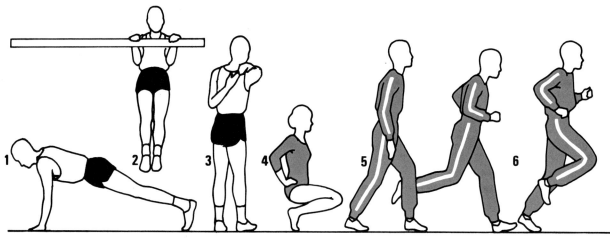

CAN YOU...

1 Do eight press-ups keeping your body straight.
2 Hang from a beam or branch and pull yourself up to look over it eight times.
3 Bend one arm up your back and the other over your shoulder behind your neck and make the fingers touch? Only score a 'yes' if you can do it both ways – first the right arm over the shoulder, then the left.
4 Do eight slow kneebends.

5 Walk four miles in under an hour.
6 Jog one mile at your own pace without feeling puffed.
7 Do any of the following: Climb several flights of stairs without becoming breathless.
Do a bout of gardening without unpleasant aches and pains.
Swim four lengths of a pool without a break.

REMEMBER WITH THE 'CAN YOU?' QUESTIONS . . . if you know you can but think it will take quite an effort mark it 'no' and don't try.

WITH THE 'DO YOU?' QUESTIONS . . . if you have any doubts about the answer, however slight, mark it 'no'.

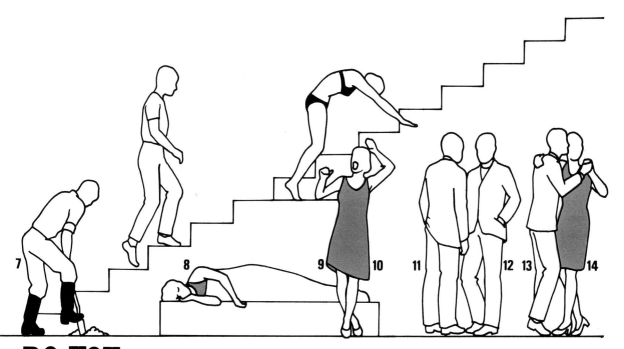

DO YOU...
8 Sleep well?
9 Wake up feeling good six mornings out of seven
10 Believe life has treated you well
11 Have friends apart from your family and work
12 Find other people ask your advice and help
13 Have a hobby or interest outside work
14 Feel you are getting the best out of life

WHY IT IS SO HARD TO BE TRULY

You meet the health challenge the moment you realise how harmful the way most of us are forced to live is **and start to do something about it.**
It is easy to forget how high the incidence of illness actually is. Certified sickness – expressed in figures for absenteeism and sick pay – has risen steadily over the last thirty years and now stands at over 400 million days per year. This figure demonstrates the difficulty so many people have with living healthily in the twentieth-century environment of rapid change and city life.
Stress illnesses – physical and mental ills caused by the daily pressures of living – are now becoming the most important causes of illness in developed countries. At its most extreme this is seen in the figures each government publishes for the causes of death, with coronary heart disease and cerebro-vascular disease topping the list. But for every person who dies of such a stress-related disease many more are sufficiently troubled to go to the doctor or take time off work. Here are some of the other illnesses that are stress-related: asthma, peptic ulcer, hiatus hernia, indigestion, bowel problems.
At the same time the incidence of 'structural' problems – backache, and so on – seems to increase in developed countries as people have tended to switch from active occupations to sedentary ones. Backache, for example, seems to be closely related to sitting down in cars or offices doing mentally stressful jobs.
Change has become the norm today. Young people about to start work or get married now **expect** to change jobs and houses quite frequently – and to move from city to city or country to country. As

well, relationships change much more rapidly than ever before. However successfully you individually may feel you cope, the fact is that generally such rapid change puts stress on our minds and bodies and this results in increased illness. One medical survey, in the United States Navy, showed clearly that sailors who had recently had significant changes in their lives, such as new jobs, relation-ships or moving home, were more prone to illness than those who led a more stable life. So health is not merely a matter of correcting the **physical** side of our lives – our nutrition, environment and exercise; medical authorities now generally accept the close health relationship between mind and body. A really healthy person tends to be someone who is 'in balance' in terms of both mind and body. Upset one and you disturb the other. Upset the mind with stress and the body responds with a physical symptom. Upset the body by depriving it of the food or exercise it needs and the mind reacts, perhaps with symptoms of nervousness or the inability to concentrate.
The person who wants to be truly healthy needs to be very aware of how almost everything he does affects his health. This is not a passport to cranky living, but a simple acceptance of the fact that health and happiness are important and worth working at. It **may** mean becoming acutely conscious of health for a period – but that is only while habits of nutrition, exercise and thinking change to match the kind of lifestyle that is likely to be healthier. Once you are healthy you won't even need to think about it, and achieving that is, above all, the superhealth challenge.

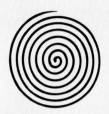

STRESS

The way many people live, especially in cities, is stressful. Women may try to raise a family and run a job at the same time. Men and women may have to commute long distances to work. All face the stress of noise, pollution, trying to improve their standard of living . . . and relationships are no longer as stable and secure as they once were.

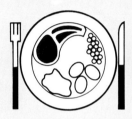

DIET

The rapid pace of life today puts pressure on people – women especially – to produce meals quickly. This has encouraged the growing use of convenience and processed foods which do not always have the nutritional value of fresh food. At the same time more of us eat in a hurry, buy quick snacks or eat between-meal fillers.

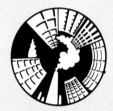

ENVIRONMENT

The urban environment in which most people live is basically unhealthy with greater air pollution, less exercise and a lack of privacy and 'space' for individuals. The rush to the country and to leisure pursuits at the weekend and during holidays reflects how unsatisfying millions of people find urban living . . . and the incidence of sickness and absenteeism shows how unhealthy it is.

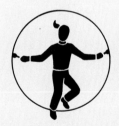

LACK OF EXERCISE

It is hard to get enough exercise in an urban environment or when your lifestyle is too full of change to accommodate regular sports or outside activities. Children are often not as fit now as their parents were at the same age and the sedentary life starts younger and younger.

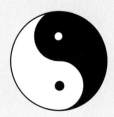

LACK OF PEACE

The body and mind need stillness and peace to 'recover' from the normal stress of daily living – especially in an urban environment. But where populations concentrate in smaller and smaller houses or flats, when leisure space is at a premium, this is increasingly hard to find.

GETTING STARTED

Ideas are one thing, acting on them is something else again – as anyone who has tried to diet or follow a programme of exercise knows. These two pages are designed to help you get started on your journey towards better health.

FIRST – Convince yourself that you want to be really healthy. Of course you are already showing an interest in your health but now you need to **convince** yourself that action is worth taking. Start by asking yourself what the real benefits of better health will be.

You will certainly **look** better. You will be more alive, more energetic, probably healthier looking. You will take a positive view of things and this also will show in the way you look. Secondly, you will probably do far more. Truly healthy people always seem to have the energy to use their time fully and to get things done. Thirdly, you will be happier because you will be more fulfilled. Finally, you will probably be more self-confident because you know, without needing someone to tell you, that you have the strength and power to decide that certain things need to be done.

NEXT – Be prepared for the hard work involved. Achieving better health may at times be the hardest thing you have ever done. This is because what you will be doing is changing some basic habits, and that is never easy. People don't like suddenly starting to walk to the station in the morning when they have driven there for years; nor do they like switching to different kinds of foods. Change is challenging; permanent change requires hard work and, sometimes, courage. You will find all sorts of excuses not to make changes. When you find yourself making them go back to the previous section and re-examine why you wanted better health in the first place. And once you've thought through a change in diet or exercise and seen it would make sense **suspect any** excuse that you then create to stop yourself doing it.

NOW – Examine your daily routines. Later we will look in detail at how daily routines and habits can create stress and ill health in our lives, and show ways of changing things for the better. The main point now is to realise that those habits which create your lifestyle are probably reinforced by routines and ways of thinking about your day which you have rarely thought about. For example, many people wrongly think they are unable to get up early in the morning because 'I'm not an early morning person'. Some **are** right, because body rhythms do vary. But many are wrong. Have you ever really put it to the test for two or three weeks? It's surprising how many women who thought they were not early morning people find that they can be when they have young children (however reluctantly at first!) And they don't go back to their late rising ways when the children are grown up. Many men whose jobs suddenly demand early rising find the same thing. We run our lives by tying ourselves to dozens of habits or ways of thinking like that. Ultimately you need to sort the good from the bad. For the moment you need to start asking how you can improve your daily routine so that you have time to exercise and time to relax in a way that really does you good.

FINALLY – Enjoy the process of gaining health. Many people take a negative attitude to improving their health, an attitude which is a sign that they **need** to improve it. They regard a programme of exercise as a difficult mountain to climb; or a change in diet as a major problem. They try to groan and moan their way to better health and, not surprisingly, often fail to get there. Better health is enjoyable and fulfilling and the process of getting there is fun. True, it's hard work too, but enjoyable hard work because you have the best possible outcome to look forward to.

It's a series of **challenges** rather than **trials,** and in meeting them you will begin to experience a whole range of feelings and thoughts which you never expected, and which are exciting. If you take up jogging for example you may, after quite a short while, feel the strange elation – some runners call it a 'high' – which many joggers feel. If you lose weight you may literally feel a new woman, or man. If you learn some of the stress control techniques we show you later you may find you can achieve much more at work or in the home than you ever believed possible. Gaining health is an enjoyable activity and a challenge to relish.

SET YOURSELF TARGETS

Management consultants sometimes recommend a simple technique for getting things done – they call it MBO, management by objectives. You set your target and a date by which you aim to achieve it and . . . off you go. And when the due date comes you assess just how far towards your target you've got. You can use a form of MBO to gain better health. You need a diary, a pencil, a couple of sheets of paper and just half an hour or so.

If you have no time to set your targets now you **can** still start by making a date with yourself to set targets. Later today? Tomorrow? At the weekend? Make an appointment with yourself, and keep it. The aim is to list some of the steps to take to start improving your health and set objectives and dates by which to achieve them. To help to keep it simple (so you don't fall into the familiar trap of spending all day in the enjoyable reverie of making a plan and then have no time to do anything about it) we show one way you might set out some health objectives with some of the options open to you in approaching each goal.

HOW TO SET YOUR FIRST TARGETS . . .

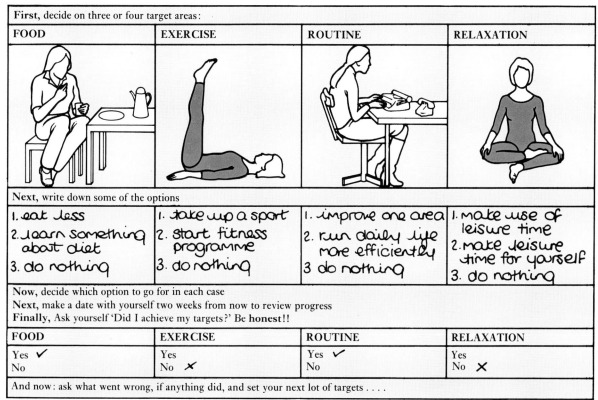

First, decide on three or four target areas:			
FOOD	EXERCISE	ROUTINE	RELAXATION

Next, write down some of the options			
1. eat less 2. learn something about diet 3. do nothing	1. take up a sport 2. start fitness programme 3. do nothing	1. improve one area 2. run daily life more efficiently 3 do nothing	1. make use of leisure time 2. make leisure time for yourself 3. do nothing

Now, decide which option to go for in each case
Next, make a date with yourself two weeks from now to review progress
Finally, Ask yourself 'Did I achieve my targets?' Be **honest**!!

FOOD	EXERCISE	ROUTINE	RELAXATION
Yes ✔ No	Yes No ✗	Yes ✔ No	Yes No ✗

And now: ask what went wrong, if anything did, and set your next lot of targets . . . .

This is only a sample of what you can do, but it should give you some pointers. It is important to set specific targets. Under the 'daily routine' section, for example, it's probably better to have as a target the improvement of one area only rather than the general target of running your life better. Always set targets you know you can achieve. Under diet, for example, it is better to aim to lose four pounds in a fortnight, because that's possible, rather than a stone, which is normally unrealistic. Success builds best on success, so your targets should be modest to begin with. As we suggest in the table, have a date about a fortnight later when you review progress, **and stick to it.** Regard it as unbreakable as an appointment with your doctor or your bank manager.

There are many ways of setting targets, and this is just one of them. The important thing is to set them, and to review progress – it's one very real way of enjoying the process of discovering wholehealth.

INTRODUCTION: THE BODYMIND

Most of us recognise in ourselves a link between our body and our mind. It occurs in all kinds of ways. A simple example, which almost everyone has experienced, is that when we have a cold we feel depressed: physical ills have mental effects. Or we may find that when we get hungry we get irritable; or when we are under a great deal of tension and stress we go down with an illness of some kind; or when we pull a muscle, strain a joint, or suffer back pain the whole world seems 'out of joint'. We call such links the Bodymind Factor.

Many women learn to recognise that at certain times of their monthly cycle they may be depressed or unbalanced in some way. At other times they may feel the opposite – on top of the world, perhaps full of sexual desire. A growing body of research suggests that men may have similar rhythms though they are harder to detect. And who hasn't fallen in love and felt their perceptions of the world change, become more clear, more wonderful? Or seen the new light and colour – health – on the face of someone in love? But while we may recognise these links between body and mind we often fail to take the next step of trying to approach our health from a 'bodymind' point of view.

HOW EXERCISE CAN HELP

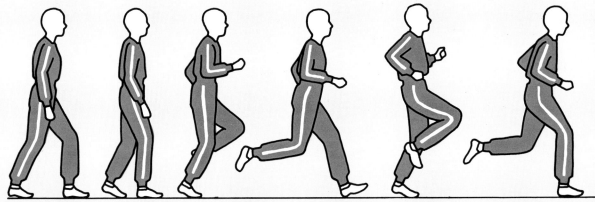

It happens every time: as a person gets physically fitter his or her mental and emotional state seems to improve. Feelings of well being, of energy, and of inner calmness seem to well up. This happens so often to people who take up regular exercise that doctors have looked for a scientific explanation – and some think they may have found it. It now seems almost certain that the key is the powerful hormone noradrenaline. This has a 'transmitter' function in the brain, and is involved in the control of impulses in the nervous system. It is produced as part of our response to stress and acts as a general stimulant to the body, increasing our alertness, concentration and ability to cope with tiredness. Too much in the system (which can occur when we are constantly under stress) appears to be damaging unless we exercise at the same time.

And it seems that the more we exercise and become generally fit the more we gain the positive benefits of this hormone. In effect, exercise helps to make us feel better.

Exercise appears to have other beneficial effects on our mental and emotional state as well. Tests in one American hospital among students suffering pre-examination nerves showed that regular jogging cut down their anxiety (and improved their marks). One side effect of exercise which also aids our mental state results from the fact that it improves our oxygen intake, which in turn oxidises a syrupy sour liquid produced in the body during muscular activity. It seems that

FACTOR

We tend to treat the symptoms rather than ask if there may be something more behind them. We treat our physical ills as something separate from our mental state – seeking medication for the symptoms, but not asking questions about the cause. Of course, the danger of asking questions about causes is that we may become amateur psychologists making problems where there are none, finding root causes that don't exist or which we don't understand. This **is** a danger, but we do not believe it is a serious one. Better to try to work out for ourselves why we get so many colds every winter and do something about it than simply to accept the fact of getting them and go on suffering for the rest of our lives. The positive aspect of such amateur psychology as this is that it may help us to approach health as a bodymind problem, that is, one which involves the whole of ourselves. In practice, the average person thinks only of the body – believing that regular jogging every morning, or any routine aimed at getting physically fit will solve health problems. But health is, if anything, more mental than physical and to achieve wholehealth you must begin to think in terms of bodymind.

This chapter aims to help you do this by showing in more detail the way in which stress, nutrition and exercise can affect your mental health; and how mental health may affect your response to all three.

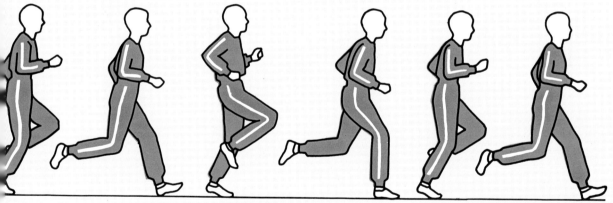

lactic acid can create a state of anxiety if introduced into the bloodstream and that levels of it rise when we are tired or under some kind of stress. By increasing our regular oxygen intake we seem more able to handle the lactic acid produced in our body.

Most of us have at some time felt the harmful effect of bottling up things inside – and the positive feelings that follow from actually **doing** something about it.

We may feel the need to shout, be violent, or simply go for a long walk by ourselves to 'calm down'. And when we've responded in one of these ways to a stressful situation we may well say 'I **feel** better for that'. How right we are, because the body's natural response to stress is physical. That's why a whole range of unconscious physical changes race through us when we are faced by danger – so we can react better to it. Too often we are unable to respond physically to stress and have to 'control ourselves', which many doctors believe may result in a harmful build-up of fatty acids in our blood vessels. Exercise helps us handle these fatty acids in a more healthy way. In Chapter 6 we show how the average unfit person (which means most people) can gradually approach exercise so that it becomes a basic part of his or her lifestyle. For the moment the main thing to understand about exercise is that you really do **feel** better for it and that's a major step towards whole health.

FOOD AND YOUR MIND

The idea that the food people eat – or **don't** eat – may be upsetting their mind and body is alien to most people: they find it hard to accept. They may feel that if they have eaten something for years it can't possibly do them harm, or that if everyone else seems to eat it without harm why shouldn't they? Or they may say that since they are not overweight, and not losing weight, that their diet **must** at least be adequate. These two pages look at the close connection between food and health, and at some of the findings that nutritionists have made which have implications for everyone.

The first thing to be clear about is that the lack of certain foods or nutrients has a direct effect on your mental state. If you take too little Vitamin B1 (thiamin) for example then you may suffer symptoms such as depression, memory lapses, loss of appetite, which are the kind of symptoms shown by some alcoholics, whose addiction can cause them to have, amongst other things, a diet too low in thiamin.

Similarly, a dietary deficiency in Vitamin B12 can cause difficulties in concentrating or memory work, and agitation. In fact B12 deficiency **does** sometimes occur among very strict vegetarians and a few individuals whose gastric juices lack intrinsic factors needed for its absorption. Such problems are most unlikely to affect you, but they demonstrate clearly that a lack of food can affect the mind as well as the body.

Equally, some research has shown that the deliberate administration of certain nutrients can improve certain mental conditions. Unfortunately

CASE HISTORY ONE A normal, bright 10-year-old girl complained of a variety of pains and headaches. Her school performance declined and she seemed less outgoing at home. She was prescribed a daily dosage of 1000 mg (1 g) of the vitamin niacin – a dosage which is far above the normal officially recommended daily intake. After four weeks the girl showed a complete recovery from her symptoms.

CASE HISTORY TWO A middle-aged woman started to be obsessive about her sheets and underclothes (which had to be perfectly ironed) and tidiness in the house. Psychoanalysis failed to produce any beneficial result. Finally, examination of her diet showed that it was unusually low in fat and protein. A change to a better diet made her far more balanced than before though it never 'cured' her – she remained nervous and inclined to get upset easily. But by sticking to the better diet she was able to control the symptoms much more easily.

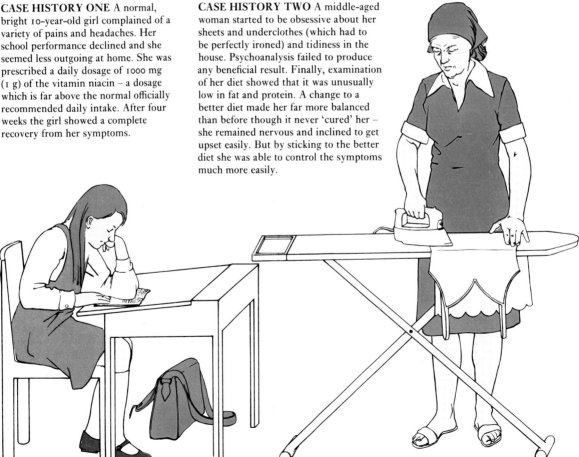

it is hard for most of us to regard individual vitamins like thiamin or niacin in terms of food, so consider instead chocolate, white flour, milk and coffee. These are foods many eat every day and which the average person would find hard to blame for mental or physical ills. Yet a growing amount of medical research suggests that hundreds of thousands of people are allergic to foods like these, and suffer physical and emotional symptoms as a result of eating them. Some of the mental symptoms of such allergies include tension, depression, overactivity and purposeless violence.

British and American doctors specialising in nutritional medicine report case after case of people with emotional disorders who can be treated and cured by a change in their diet.

Significantly from the point of view of the mind/body link, many of these cases display physical *and* mental symptoms.

One well-documented area where a dietary problem produces emotional symptoms is hypoglycaemia – a deficiency of sugar in the blood. If for some reason a person's blood fails to carry sufficient glucose to the brain a variety of symptoms can occur: nervousness, depression or weeping for no obvious reason.

The following three case histories demonstrate the kind of effects a change in diet can have on the mental health of individual patients.

CASE HISTORY THREE Fear of enclosed spaces (claustrophobia) and depression were the symptoms of one young man treated successfully by nutritional medicine. Analysis of what he ate showed that, like many people, his diet was unbalanced – in his case it consisted almost exclusively of hamburgers and black coffee. This had resulted in a deterioration in the ability of his body to produce energy. A change to a better diet was slow to work because his body was unable to absorb nutrients easily. But extra vitamin therapy and patience with the improved diet was eventually successful and the claustrophobia disappeared.

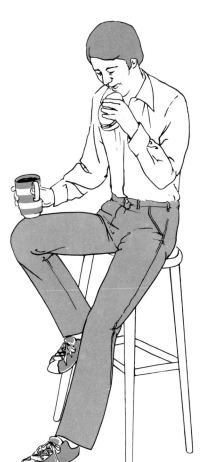

Cases like these, which occur frequently in nutritional medicine literature, have little value in helping us individually to find health – the information given is too slight. Their main value lies in under-lining the importance of diet as a factor in our mental as well as physical health. This is something we easily forget – even though we might experience it positively when we go on a **good** successful diet and feel better for it, or when we feel the emotional after effects of eating food that does not 'agree' with us.

In Chapter 4 we look in more detail at the contribution different foods and nutrients make to our health; and in Chapters 7 and 8 at how to achieve a healthy diet.

The main point now to realise is that you don't have to be a food faddist to be interested in your food. In fact NOT to be interested is as shortsighted as the man who fills his car's petrol tank from a can with no label on it – and never bothers to find out if he might be pouring in washing-up liquid rather than petrol. But that is how shortsighted most people still are about their diet.

YOUR BODY RHYTHMS

We all sense that our physical stamina and emotional state fluctuate so that we have good times and bad. Times when we say 'Everything's gone wrong today and I really feel under the weather', or 'I've been so full of energy today it has been incredible.' Women recognise such rhythms, and learn to live with them far better than men because they have the tangible evidence of their menstrual cycle. But men have emotional and physical rhythms too, as research by Danish, British and Japanese doctors and psychologists has shown. The levels of sex hormones in the urine of men, for example, appear to fluctuate on a monthly basis; and industrial psychologists have charted emotional ups and downs of male workers and found they fall into a cyclical pattern. We often acknowledge some of the rhythms by which our bodies appear to function without realising it.

Take something as apparently unrelated to rhythms as the time at which most Western people drink alcohol. It's acceptable to have a sociable drink or two at 7 o'clock in the evening, socially unacceptable to have exactly the same drink in the morning. A team of doctors in the University of Minnesota in America injected mice with the equivalent of a quarter bottle of vodka **at different times of their day** to see if the effects varied. They did: dramatically. Nearly two thirds died if it was administered at their normal awakening time, only 12 per cent died if it was administered at the start of a rest period. Many people are aware that alcohol affects them differently at different times of the day. Many executives, for example, who need to be mentally active in the afternoon will refuse to drink much at lunch-time because 'it makes me so sleepy'. Yet the same drink in the evening may not affect them the same way.

Does any of this matter? And what is its relevance to better health? The short answers to these questions are 'Yes' and 'Quite a lot'. There is increasing evidence that when people are ill their normal rhythms become unsynchronised. For example, those with liver ailments often have a peak in temperature and urination at night, instead of (as normal) in the morning.

A study comparing the daily changes in temperature, potassium excretion, urine flow and heart rate in a group of patients suffering depression and in normal patients suggested that the potassium excretion was out of tune with urine flow among the depressed patients. Similar correlations between illness and disruption of internal metabolic rhythms have been widely observed by doctors.

It suggests that when we are healthy our rhythms are in tune, when we are not they are not. And, as ever, our language unconsciously acknowledges such patterns – 'He's mixed up', 'she's not in tune with herself' or 'he's such a balanced individual'. When we use such phrases of others we are really commenting on their health and accepting that rhythms and health do go together.

In practice we disrupt or ignore our daily and monthly rhythms at our own peril. Long-distance air travellers know the problem of jet-lag too well – when their judgement appears to be suspect for a period after their journey is over and they arrive somewhere during the day while their body is still (as at home) thinking it is night. Many firms now insist that their travelling executives take a day's rest after a long air journey before starting business.

Research into the work ability and illness rates among night and shift workers suggests that a change from normal day-night-day rhythms can be damaging. Meter readers in a Swedish gasworks, for example, make more mistakes at night; industrial accidents occur more frequently in the small hours of the morning; telephone and radar operators work less effectively at times when they would normally be asleep.

If we accept the importance of rhythms the next step is to ask if there is anything we can do about them: how can we measure our own rhythms?

We may not be able to analyse our own blood or urine for chemical changes but we **can** be much more observant of ourselves. We can begin to see how our feelings of hunger vary, when we get cold, when we feel most alive, when we are most sensitive to colour, smell or touch, and even when our digestion seems to work best. We can watch our monthly changes and try to accommodate them into our lifestyles. We may even find that biorhythmic charts help us to watch ourselves better.

In effect we can become more sensitive to our minds and body – to ourselves – and that is a real step to being more healthy.

DAILY RHYTHMS

Many rhythms of life run close to the twenty-four hour day we normally keep, as you would expect when so much is determined by the rhythm of the sun. Our body temperature, for example, rises and falls rhythmically through the day, reaching a low point normally early in the morning. But individuals vary, some finding their temperature rising fast in the morning, others being relatively sluggish.

Immunity to infection appears to be related to the blood level of gamma globulin (a serum containing most immune antibodies to viruses). The level of this fluctuates daily, being at its lowest at night when we are normally asleep and isolated from others. Perhaps this accounts for the extra colds and infections often suffered by students studying late for examinations, shift workers, and long-distance air travellers. Our sensory perception, ability to perform demanding mental tasks and physical co-ordination change through the day. Many athletes now vary their training schedules to fit their physical rhythms. Most of us have an awareness that we perform well at certain times of the day, perhaps regarding ourselves as 'larks' or 'owls'.

HOW TEMPERATURE VARIES THROUGH THE DAY IN A TYPICAL PERSON

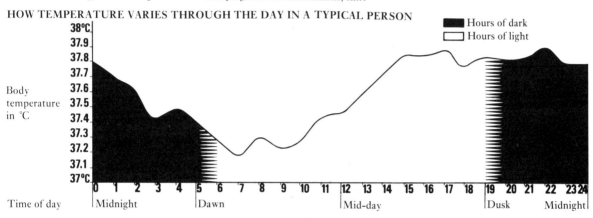

■ Hours of dark
□ Hours of light

Body temperature in °C

Time of day — Midnight | Dawn | Mid-day | Dusk | Midnight

MONTHLY RHYTHMS

These are perhaps harder to account for, though they are as well established as daily rhythms. Indeed they have become almost a popular fad in the form of computerised biorhythms which chart what are believed to be (by their supporters) three fundamental human cycles – intellectual (33 days), emotional (28 days) and physical (23 days). The idea is that each cycle starts at birth and since they have a different length there may be days when we are very low or high on each cycles, average days and 'changeover' days when one or more of the cycles is shifting from an active to a passive phase, or the reverse.

Research on personnel in the United States Navy appears to confirm the validity of these ideas, and they have been applied successfully to fields as varied as teaching, industrial safety and athletic performance. It is worth pointing out, however, that many people who have examined biorhythms have found no easy correlation between them and their normal lives. However this does not disprove the idea but merely confirms what scientists interested in human rhythms already know – that we vary individually a great deal and no simple 'rhythm rules' for everyone can be devised.

BIORHYTHMS

■ Intellectual energy
●● Emotional energy
▬ Physical energy

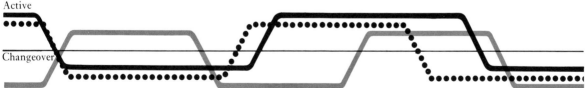

February | March

Active

Changeover

Passive

A typical biorhythmic chart reading showing an individual's intellectual, emotional and physical energies. The chart shows that this person will be very active on all fronts in the middle of March, very passive at the end of March and going through a difficult changeover period in the third week of February. The chart suggests that February 20–27 is a good period to get on with physical jobs like decorating, or perhaps start a new sport, while March 8–12 is an excellent period to think through problems, come up with solutions but not to do anything about them quite yet . . .

THE STRESS FACTOR 1

Dr Thomas Holmes, Professor of Psychiatry at the University of Washington, has estimated that four out of every five people who experience dramatic changes in their lives can expect to suffer a major illness within two years of the change. With another researcher, Richard Rahe, he actually put figures to the importance of different stress factors which help underline the way in which 'normal' life changes may be contributors to our ill health. Few things demonstrate better the interdependence of mind and body than our physical responses to mental stress. Every one of us has seen – and

personally suffered from – the way in which a mental pressure creates a physical response. A scolding from our mother makes us cry; sudden danger makes us shake with fear; real anger may make us strike out without thinking about the consequences. We are so used to such causes and effects that we incorporate our often instinctive understanding of them into the way we respond to others. When we ask a friend who is white faced and tired, 'Aren't you **feeling** well?' we acknowledge our unspoken understanding of the link between the mind and body.

STRESS VALUE OF LIFE CHANGES
If you relate this table to your life over the last year and score more than 150 then you are under some stress and you have a fifty-fifty chance of suffering illness. This does not mean you will get ill, merely that there is a greater chance you will.

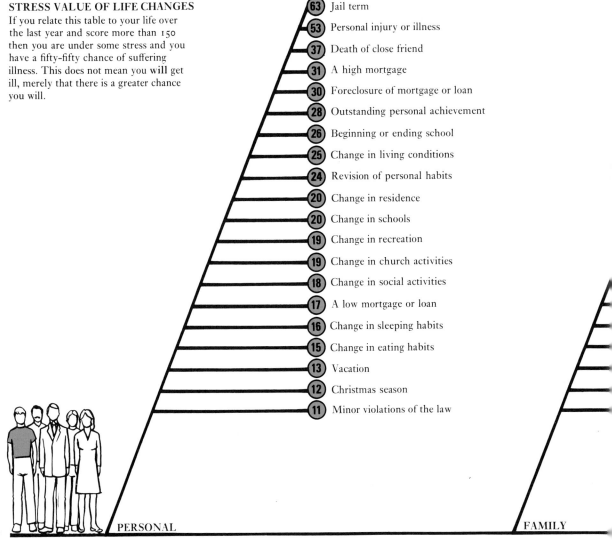

- **63** Jail term
- **53** Personal injury or illness
- **37** Death of close friend
- **31** A high mortgage
- **30** Foreclosure of mortgage or loan
- **28** Outstanding personal achievement
- **26** Beginning or ending school
- **25** Change in living conditions
- **24** Revision of personal habits
- **20** Change in residence
- **20** Change in schools
- **19** Change in recreation
- **19** Change in church activities
- **18** Change in social activities
- **17** A low mortgage or loan
- **16** Change in sleeping habits
- **15** Change in eating habits
- **13** Vacation
- **12** Christmas season
- **11** Minor violations of the law

PERSONAL

FAMILY

When we have distressing news for people – really bad news – we may ask them to sit down before telling them what it is because we know it is more physically stressful for them to 'take it' standing up. When we see people fidgeting or looking troubled we know that 'something is on their mind'. What we are slower to acknowledge is the effect that the many different stresses inherent in our own particular lifestyle may be having on our bodies – and our health. It is worth looking at this problem in more detail because it affects us directly, and through the harm stress does to our families and friends.

For millions of people, particularly the majority of us who live and work in crowded towns and cities, the stress factors are the same: noise, polluted air, job competition, difficult relationships, visual overstimulation . . . the list seems endless. Some of these factors – like job competition – create mental stress, others – like long-distance commuting – are physical. Both are important, but here we concentrate on mental stress because it is not so well recognised by most people as a real danger to their health.

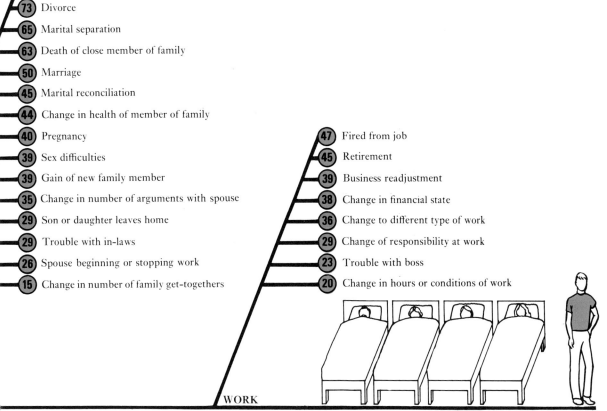

- **100** Death of spouse
- **73** Divorce
- **65** Marital separation
- **63** Death of close member of family
- **50** Marriage
- **45** Marital reconciliation
- **44** Change in health of member of family
- **40** Pregnancy
- **39** Sex difficulties
- **39** Gain of new family member
- **35** Change in number of arguments with spouse
- **29** Son or daughter leaves home
- **29** Trouble with in-laws
- **26** Spouse beginning or stopping work
- **15** Change in number of family get-togethers

- **47** Fired from job
- **45** Retirement
- **39** Business readjustment
- **38** Change in financial state
- **36** Change to different type of work
- **29** Change of responsibility at work
- **23** Trouble with boss
- **20** Change in hours or conditions of work

WORK

THE STRESS FACTOR 2

Why should this be so? How is it that mental stresses should have physical results? The answers lie within the actual experience of each of us. Think back to when you were last suddenly put in a stressful situation **which went on for a long time.** (It may be that you are in such a situation now.) Perhaps it was coping with examinations, perhaps moving house; maybe it was a sustained argument with someone or working against a deadline at the office. If you think about your response to these situations you will probably find that it goes through three stages:
– First you get ready to meet the challenge, your reactions speeding up and your strength growing.
– Next you meet the challenge, handling it better for having mobilised yourself to do so.
– But finally as it goes on and on you begin to get tired and perhaps feel you can't cope. Perhaps physical symptoms like a headache, aching shoulders, a cold, set in.
This is a very generalised description of reaction to prolonged stress but it probably has familiar elements in it for you.
It is when the third stage goes on too long as the stress factor becomes prolonged that it begins to take its toll on you physically. This is because when we react to mental stress we tend to over-react physically, a reminder that we were

once animals who had to learn to flee danger or fight it. The executive faced by a crisis will never have to fight physically, or actually flee – but his body behaves as if he did have to as his pulse races, his blood pressure rises, and his muscles are fuelled with sugar and fatty acids by hormonal changes. Living a continually stressed life like this can have a wide range of physical effects, some of them fatal. Heart attacks are more common among the highly stressed because the heart cannot cope with a continual high rate and high blood pressure. Such people often have resources to drugs like alcohol and nicotine as a release but these appear to increase the internal physical conditions which are a prelude to a heart attack. High-stress people suffer stomach ulcers or colitis – inflammation of the colon. Or we may choose another option – to try to hide from it. From a health point of view both may be damaging. By suffering stress continually we exhaust ourselves mentally and physically and become vulnerable to ill health – as is shown by statistics of stress-related diseases among people living under pressure. But if we switch off we are effectively putting blinkers on ourselves, shutting off whole areas of sensitivity to sight, touch, smell and sound. Look at the faces of the average group of commuters travelling to work surrounded by stresses of all kinds – they are often

expressionless, half dead. Many will fall asleep or use a newspaper or book to hide behind. What they are doing – and at some time most of us have done it – makes a lot of sense at that particular moment. But its long-term effect may be to reduce the ways in which we allow ourselves to be stimulated by things around us. Although many deny that this happens to **them** the moment they are put into a non-stressful situation and invited to feel new sensations – the classic situation is a class in yoga but the same applies to a city family at the seaside for a day – they feel their awareness expanding in all kinds of directions. Life suddenly seems much happier and more exciting. They are exploring outside themselves, rather than hiding inside themselves.
And in this situation there can be little doubt that people come nearer to wholehealth: they find they have more energy to do things; their sex life may be much better on holiday than back at home; they are more relaxed too about things that go wrong.
In effect, the health of their mind and body improves until the stress situation returns. But suffering OR switching off are not the only ways of coping with stress. A third is to cut out habits which create stress and adopt others which reduce it. This is what achieving better health involves, and what many of the sections in this book will help you do.

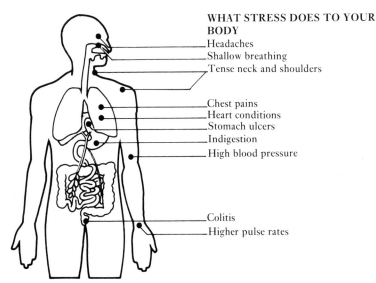

WHAT STRESS DOES TO YOUR BODY
Headaches
Shallow breathing
Tense neck and shoulders

Chest pains
Heart conditions
Stomach ulcers
Indigestion
High blood pressure

Colitis
Higher pulse rates

INTRODUCTION

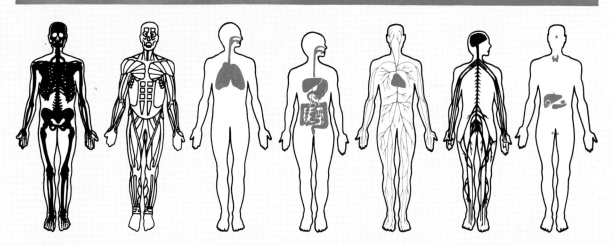

APPRECIATE YOUR BODY – THE FIRST STEP TO HEALTH

Really healthy people **look** as if they're healthy: their colour is good, they move well, and they seem at ease with their bodies – and themselves. And while they are rarely self-conscious about the way they look, they are often very conscious of what their body says to them. Just as a good gardener or cook knows naturally what's needed, a truly healthy person knows too. Living healthily – and how you do that varies with every individual – becomes a natural way of life.

But just as gardeners and cooks need to learn their skill, so do people often need to learn to respond to their own physical needs. For many people, reared in cultural traditions which tend to constrict natural physical expression and make it self-conscious, this can be hard. Especially when the word 'health' is associated more with ill health and its symptoms than a natural celebration of life. If you are one of the millions of people who have never felt fully healthy, one of the first steps you can take to feeling good is to appreciate what you've already got. For your body – however unhealthy, flabby, weak, or plain it may sometimes feel – is a marvellous creation which you probably can learn to **enjoy** much more than you do. One way to start doing this is to know something of how it works. That's why in the section that follows we look at the body not as a mass of cells, or a collection of different organs, but as a series of perfectly integrated systems.

You must know how your body works (pages 24–25)
The Skeletal system – your body's inner scaffolding (pages 26–27)
The Muscular system – for conscious and unconscious movement (pages 28–29)
The Breathing system – the breath of life (pages 30–31)
The Digestive system – how your body processes food (pages 32–33)
Blood circulation – your body's road system (pages 34–35)
Urinary and Liver system – processing and the body's waste disposal system (pages 36–37)
The Reproductive system – (pages 38–39)
The nervous system (pages 40–41)
Metabolism (pages 42–43)

YOU MUST KNOW HOW YOUR BODY

All of us are different but the basic systems on which we depend are the same. Your **skeletal system** gives you the inner scaffolding you need for support and movement, combining with your **muscles** to make conscious movement and reflex processes possible.

Your **respiratory system** brings oxygen into your body and also disposes of some waste products. Oxygen and nutrients are transported internally by the **circulatory system** whose central organ is

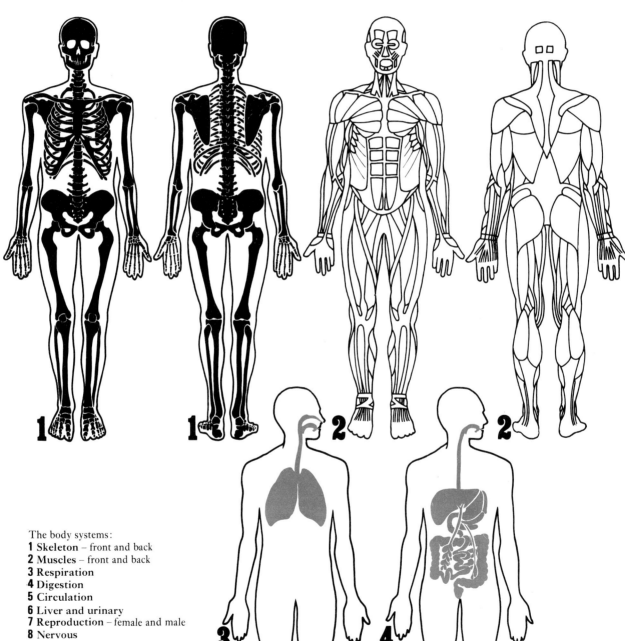

The body systems:
1 Skeleton – front and back
2 Muscles – front and back
3 Respiration
4 Digestion
5 Circulation
6 Liver and urinary
7 Reproduction – female and male
8 Nervous
9 Metabolism and endocrine

WORKS

the heart. Your **digestive system** processes what you eat, much of the waste being disposed of by the **urinary system,** while **reproduction** makes new life, and evolution, possible. Controlling it all is the **nervous system,** the link between your brain and your body, the **endocrine system,** which uses hormones as its agents, and **metabolism,** the chemical regulation of the body.

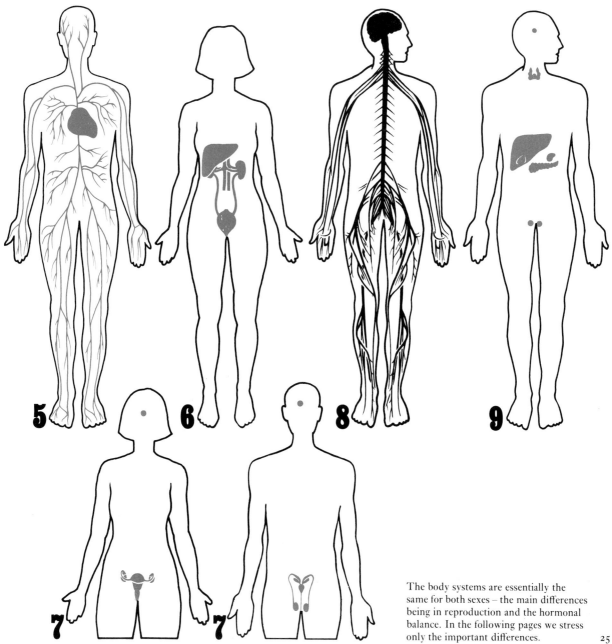

The body systems are essentially the same for both sexes – the main differences being in reproduction and the hormonal balance. In the following pages we stress only the important differences.

25

THE SKELETAL SYSTEM

Only when something goes wrong with one of the bones and joints that make up the body's inner scaffolding do you realise just how important it is to you. Sprain an ankle, get tennis elbow, put a disc out in your back and it affects the whole of the rest of you. The skeleton has three jobs – it supports the body along with the muscles; it protects vital organs like the brain, heart and lungs; and it makes movement possible. It is a wonderful example of precision engineering which combines great strength – some of the bones are as strong as steel – with balance and flexibility. Man's hands have a wider range of movement than any other animal. At birth there are about 350 separate bones in the body, but as growth occurs many of these fuse until there are just over 200 when the body stops growing in the early twenties. The bones themselves rarely go wrong, although a vitamin D deficiency will cause rickets in children and osteomalacia (weak, brittle bones) in adults. But most problems arise when ligaments, tendons and muscles weaken through bad posture and allow bones to move out of position.

AXIAL

At first glance a skeleton looks like a jumble of bones with little order, but it is not hard to make sense of it. Start with the skull, spine and ribcage, these form the **axial** skeleton – the central part of the system. The skull's main job is to protect the brain. It is made up of twenty-nine bones joined together to form a single unit, except for the lower jawbone which can move independently and makes chewing possible. Most important structurally is the spine, made up of thirty-three vertebrae. The first seven are called the cervical vertebrae, making up the neck. The first two of these – the atlas and the axis – are cleverly designed joints which give your head considerable range of movement, allowing you to look sideways, down at the ground and upwards. Below these lie the twelve thoracic vertebrae, forming the upper back. From them the twelve pairs of ribs curve out and round to the front to form the chest, making a protective cage for the heart and lungs. The five lumbar vertebrae below these form the small of the back, followed by five sacral vertebrae (fused together and inflexible) and a final four forming the coccyx, which is virtually one bone. The discs between each vertebra and the strong muscles that run up either side combine to give the spine great strength and shock-absorbing powers.

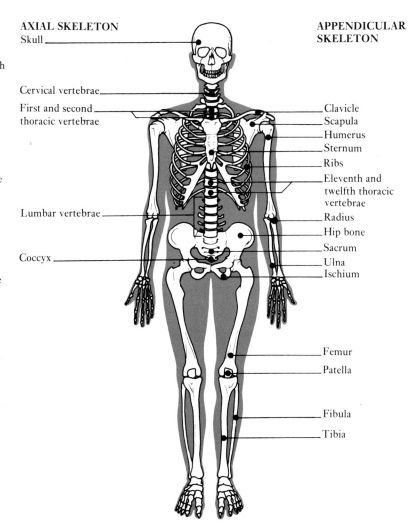

AXIAL SKELETON

Skull

Cervical vertebrae

First and second thoracic vertebrae

Lumbar vertebrae

Coccyx

APPENDICULAR SKELETON

Clavicle
Scapula
Humerus
Sternum
Ribs
Eleventh and twelfth thoracic vertebrae
Radius
Hip bone
Sacrum
Ulna
Ischium
Femur
Patella
Fibula
Tibia

BONES

There are four types of bones in the body, their shape and composition reflecting their different jobs. There are long tubular bones (the limbs); short bones of fibrous tissue (the wrist and ankle); flat, plate-like bones (those making up the skull); and irregular bones like the vertebrae and those in the face. The biggest is the thigh bone (femur), the smallest are the tiny ossicles in the inner ear, fractions of an inch in size.

APPENDICULAR

The second part of the skeletal system is the **appendicular** skeleton – the pectoral girdle (shoulders), the limbs and the pelvic girdle. Look at the ingenious way in which the pectoral girdle fits over the ribcage joining with the sternum in front and the spine at the back. Its two clavicles give support for the shoulders, themselves formed of the two scapulae. All of this gives a point of leverage for the two arms. It is a surprisingly light structure considering the heavy work the shoulders and arms often tackle. The pelvic girdle, which transmits the weight of the trunk of the body to the legs, is a much heavier structure. It is formed from the sacrum and the two hip bones, the ilium and ischium. The pelvic girdle supports the lower abdomen and associated organs and provides a base for each of the massive thigh bones (femur) to fit into.

The hip is probably the most heavily worked joint in the body. The pelvic girdle joins the femur (above), and the fibula and tibia (below) join the femur at the knee with the protective kneecap (patella) moving freely in front of it. And don't forget the feet – each foot is made up of twenty-six bones – between them they have a quarter of the bones in the body.

BONE STRUCTURE

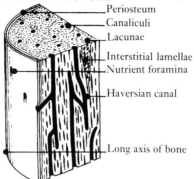

- Periosteum
- Canaliculi
- Lacunae
- Interstitial lamellae
- Nutrient foramina
- Haversian canal
- Long axis of bone

BONE MATERIAL

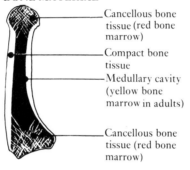

- Cancellous bone tissue (red bone marrow)
- Compact bone tissue
- Medullary cavity (yellow bone marrow in adults)
- Cancellous bone tissue (red bone marrow)

CARTILAGE

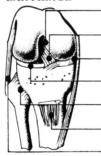

The knee
- Posterior cruciate ligament
- Anterior cruciate ligament
- Medial meniscus (Semilunar cartilage)
- Lateral meniscus (Semilunar cartilage)
- Tibio-fibular ligament
- Ligamentum patellae
- Fibular collateral ligament

FONTANELLES

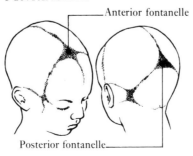

- Anterior fontanelle
- Posterior fontanelle

How it's made

Bones are not dry, dead material – one third of them is living tissue with a constant turnover of cells carrying out the jobs of maintenance and repair. Bones are serviced by blood vessels, nerves and lymph vessels (transporting body fluids) which run through a labyrinth of tiny canals.

Special cells (osteoblasts) can carry out repair work on bones while others (osteoclasts) can dissolve and break down damaged bones so that they can be repaired.

What it is

Bones develop from cartilage (which makes up the softer, lighter framework of many bones). This ossifies due to a build-up of different minerals, eventually forming a hard outer shell. Children's bones are composed of two-thirds cartilage and one-third mineral compound, giving them lightness, suppleness and the ability to grow. Adult bones are mainly mineral compound and so are heavier and stronger, growing brittle in later years.

What it's for

Cartilage, which forms organs like the outer ear and epiglottis, is bonelike but is formed of two protein materials, collagen (the harder of the two) and elastin (more springy). Fibrocartilage (containing more collagen and so harder) forms spinal discs, while hyalin is the hard bluish material found at the end of of bones, and linking the ribs and breastbone. Tendons link muscle to bone, ligaments link bones to each other.

Why they are needed

The bones of the cranium of a newborn child are separated by six gaps called fontanelles, each protected by membrane. These give the skull flexibility for delivery at birth and allow for growth. But they make a child's skull very vulnerable until they ossify in the second year. However, they do not fully harden until maturity, allowing for the continued growth of the brain.

THE MUSCULAR SYSTEM

Your body would literally collapse without muscles. They make it possible for you to move, stand or sit, and also for your heart, stomach and other areas to function. They make up two-fifths of the body's weight – ranging from the largest in your buttocks used for walking or climbing stairs, to the smallest, in your ear.

There are 620 **voluntary** muscles – those over which you have control. They are often called the skeletal muscles because, in the main, they are attached to the skeleton. Under a microscope they have a striped appearance due to the way they are made. A series of bundles of fibres with protein at their core, they have the ability to contract very fast when they receive an impulse from the brain telling them to do so. But they cannot forcefully expand, which explains why you have two muscles in your arms, the triceps and biceps – one pulling your forearm forward, the other pulling it back, each doing its work by contracting.

A second group of muscles, controlling the movement of the intestines, blood vessels, uterus and most other internal organs, are called involuntary because we have no conscious control over them. They are made from a smoother material which moves with wavelike motions. Their muscle fibres run along the muscle and across them giving them the ability to work in two directions.

The heart is a muscle on its own – it is striated like the skeletal muscles and very powerful, but we have no conscious control over it. Certain situations like fear or danger can affect the speed

THE DIFFERENT MUSCLES

The body is covered by a mass of interwoven muscles which give it support, shape and movement. We are aware of only a few of them. The **masseter,** for example, links the cheekbone and the lower jaw and makes chewing possible. Clench your teeth and you can feel it bunch in the angle of the jaw. The **trapezius** runs from the head down the back of the neck to the shoulders and pulls the head back. The **intercostals** link the ribs, expanding and contracting the ribcage as we breathe. If we are stressed they may tense up, causing pains in the chest. The **deltoids** form the rounded 'corner' between shoulder and arms and lift the arms from the body. The complex back muscles, dominated by the **latissimus dorsi,** give it enormous strength and flexibility. The massive **gluteus maximus,** the main buttock muscle, links the ilium and femur bones. The thigh is made up of several muscles, the main one of which is the **rectus femoris** running in the front from hip to knee, which straightens the leg at the knee when it contracts. Finally, the familiar calf muscle is called the gastrocnemius, one of a group of three down the back of the lower leg.

FRONT

BACK

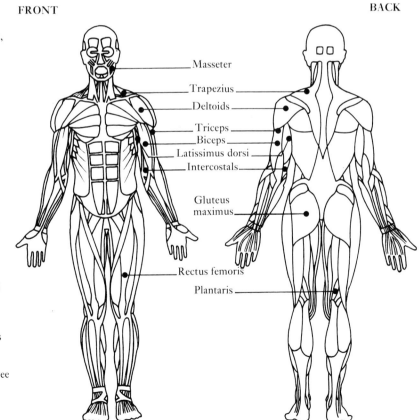

Masseter
Trapezius
Deltoids
Triceps
Biceps
Latissimus dorsi
Intercostals
Gluteus maximus
Rectus femoris
Plantaris

at which the heart beats – the increased heart rate associated with fear being a mechanism to provide other muscles with the oxygen they need (transported by the blood) to go into rapid motion if need for rapid action arises.

But the muscles we are most aware of are the skeletal muscles for we know immediately if they are strained or tired. These are the ones that do heavy work for us, sometimes at great speed: they make it possible for us to run for a bus, lift heavy suitcases, or delicately cut out an intricate shape in paper. The fuel they burn as they work is glucose, carried to them by the blood, which is why some athletes eat glucose to help their performance. As the glucose is used there is a build-up of water, carbon dioxide, lactic acid and heat – as anyone who has ever done a heavy job

knows. As lactic acid builds up, the muscle finds it harder to contract and we feel fatigued. Only oxygen can clear the lactic acid away, which is why we breathe faster and our hearts pump more blood when we are active. It may take some time to pay off this oxygen debt before we recover from strenuous activity – so we continue to pant, and our heart beats fast for a while after stopping the activity. For fit people this recovery period is much shorter, nor do they feel muscle fatigue nearly as quickly as the unfit. Even when we are asleep the voluntary muscles are active, maintaining a weak contraction and their 'tone' or ability to act immediately they are needed.

HOW MUSCLES WORK

Because muscles can only **contract** with force, you need one muscle group to raise a limb and another to lower it. In the arm the brachialis **raises** the lower arm by contracting, while the triceps relaxes; when the triceps **lowers** the forearm, the brachialis relaxes. Try contracting both at once so that they go hard simultaneously – you won't be able to do it! Muscles at most of the joints in the body are arranged in opposing pairs like this.

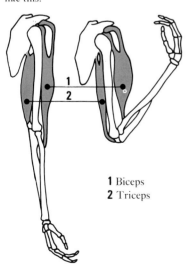

1 Biceps
2 Triceps

FROWNING – SMILING

The human face has a wide range of expressions due to the thirty or more muscles linking facial skin to skull. You frown when the orbicularis and corrugator muscles contract; you smile when the zygomaticus and orbicularis combine to narrow the eyes and pull the mouth back and up.

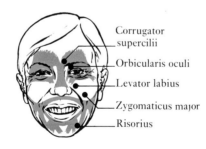

Corrugator supercilii
Orbicularis oculi
Levator labius
Zygomaticus major
Risorius

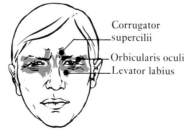

Corrugator supercilii
Orbicularis oculi
Levator labius

CRAMP

This is the painful spasmodic contraction of muscles, usually in the limbs, especially the calf, thigh or feet.

Most people know instinctively what to do when they suffer cramp – they rub, grasp, massage or stroke the affected part to stimulate the nerves. This should be done gently at first as being too rough may aggravate the condition. Moving the limb back and forth if it is cramp in the leg, foot or arm often helps as well. Indeed, when a cramp starts coming on, it may be possible to avoid it by moving the limb, or massaging it.

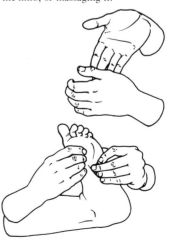

THE BREATHING SYSTEM

Everyone knows the physical and mental joy of taking a really deep breath of fresh air. More than any other physical process, breathing **feels** like life itself.

It makes you feel good because it is the body's way of constantly rejuvenating itself by taking in fresh oxygen and getting rid of carbon dioxide and water.

This exchange of gases takes place in minute air sacs in the lungs but before it even gets there the air has been cleaned and warmed to body temperature by an ingenious process starting in the nose.

Large dust particles are removed from the air as it enters the nose by the coarse nasal hairs. Behind the nose there are moist, glistening membranes which trap more dust. This mucous membrane has microscopic hairlike structures (cilia) which propel the dust and bacteria caught down into the throat where it is swallowed.

At the same time the air has been warmed and it passes into the pharynx – situated behind the nose and mouth. Here the air goes past the tonsils and adenoids and down into the windpipe (trachea). Here it passes through the larynx, a small, box-shaped structure of muscles protected by cartilage supporting the vocal cords which vibrate when air is forced through them.

At the entrance to the trachea is a protective device, the epiglottis, which basically prevents food particles entering the trachea and choking you when you swallow.

Like the mucous membrane the trachea is also covered with cilia which carry bacteria and dust

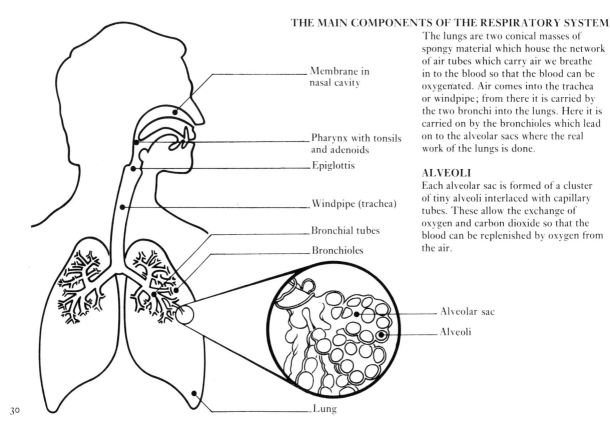

THE MAIN COMPONENTS OF THE RESPIRATORY SYSTEM

The lungs are two conical masses of spongy material which house the network of air tubes which carry air we breathe in to the blood so that the blood can be oxygenated. Air comes into the trachea or windpipe; from there it is carried by the two bronchi into the lungs. Here it is carried on by the bronchioles which lead on to the alveolar sacs where the real work of the lungs is done.

ALVEOLI

Each alveolar sac is formed of a cluster of tiny alveoli interlaced with capillary tubes. These allow the exchange of oxygen and carbon dioxide so that the blood can be replenished by oxygen from the air.

Membrane in nasal cavity

Pharynx with tonsils and adenoids

Epiglottis

Windpipe (trachea)

Bronchial tubes

Bronchioles

Alveolar sac

Alveoli

Lung

away from the lungs. The cleaned and warmed air enters the two lungs through the bronchial tubes. These subdivide into bronchioles and in turn into millions of tiny air sacs called alveoli.

It is here that the lungs' job is carried out. Each alveolus is made of a delicate membrane structure of cells strengthened by elastic fibres of tissues and interlaced with capillary vessels. These transport de-oxygenated blood carrying carbon dioxide from the pulmonary artery and takes fresh blood to the the pulmonary veins to be pumped round into the heart and then round the arteries.

The trigger for each breath (and for increasing the rate of breathing) is the level of acidity in the blood measured by the amount of carbon dioxide in it. This sets off a brain impulse to set the muscles moving. This sensitive mechanism makes sure that we always get enough oxygen. It comes into play when you try to hold your breath for too long and you suddenly start gulping for air. This is why it would never be possible to kill yourself voluntarily by holding your breath – the involuntary breathing impulses would take over and start you breathing again.

There are other protective reactions associated with breathing. We cough and sneeze when dust enters the air passages of the lungs or nose as a way of getting rid of it quickly. Hiccupping, often caused by indigestion, occurs when the diaphragm contracts spasmodically, causing sudden breathing which causes the vocal cords to close tight with the familiar 'hiccup' sound.

INWARD BREATH
Diaphragm falls – air enters

OUTWARD BREATH
Diaphragm rises – air expelled

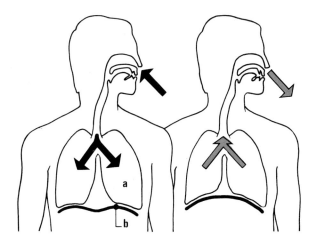

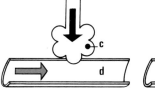

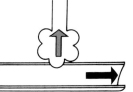

a Lungs
b Diaphragm
c Air sac
d Capillaries
➡ Oxygen
➩ Carbon dioxide

HOW WE BREATHE IN AND OUT

Breathing occurs as a result of muscular effort. The key muscle is the broad curved diaphragm at the base of the ribcage. When it contracts the volume of the lungs increases, drawing air into the space created. When it relaxes the lungs partially collapse, pressure increases and air is driven out.

The movement of the lungs is three-dimensional. The ribs (the protective cages of bones around the lungs) are hinged to the spine and linked to the breastbone. All the components move at once, allowing the constant expansion and contraction necessary for breathing. We breathe in and out about sixteen times a minute, taking in about one pint of air by volume each time. This can be greatly increased when necessary. In fact, we can breathe about twenty times as much when active than when at rest – the maximum intake being around 5 pints.

Oxygen and carbon dioxide are exchanged between the walls of the air sacs and capillaries – the oxygen goes into the blood and the carbon dioxide to the lungs before being breathed out.

THE DIGESTIVE SYSTEM

We eat to live. But what we eat must be broken down into molecules before the body can absorb the parts it needs for energy, repair and building. This is what the digestive system does by putting food through a series of mechanical, chemical and temperature changes as it passes down the alimentary canal – the passage from the mouth to the anus.

The process starts even before you eat. The thought or sight of food makes your mouth water, and this saliva contains enzymes which begin the chemical breakdown.

Food passes from the mouth to the oesophagus with a conscious swallow but after that the body takes over with automatic waves of contraction which push the food down to the stomach.

An adult's stomach can hold about $2\frac{1}{2}$ pints and will take three-to-five hours to process the food – churning and squeezing it to mix it with the gastric juices released in the stomach.

These juices contain enzymes – chemical agents which act on the food and convert it into fatty acids, glycerol and sugars which can be used for repair or energy in the body.

Further muscular contractions squeeze the partly digested food into the duodenum – the foot-long tube connecting the stomach with the small intestine. Complex reactions between the body and various foods release different hormones which regulate the juices acting on the foods, and the speed at which it is processed. So foods that are harder to digest, like proteins, move more slowly through the system. The liver has an important accessory role in some of these processes.

By the time the food leaves the duodenum to enter the small intestine – 'small' because of its width rather than its length which is over 20 feet – it has been broken down by the acids and enzymes into a creamy fluid called chyme.

THE DIGESTIVE TRACT

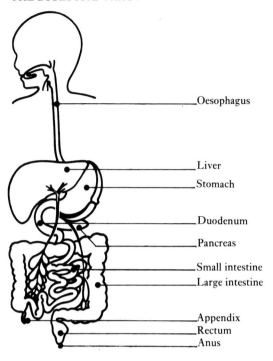

Oesophagus

Liver
Stomach

Duodenum

Pancreas

Small intestine
Large intestine

Appendix
Rectum
Anus

THE DIGESTIVE PROCESS

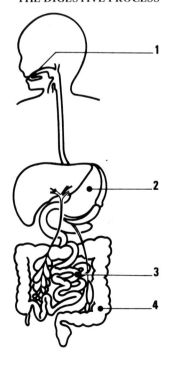

Digestion starts in the mouth (**1**) where saliva starts breaking down starch. Pepsis in the stomach (**2**) starts digestion of protein although most protein is absorbed in the small intestine (**3**). Here too the fats are emulsified in a series of complex chemical changes which end with fats passing into the lymph vessels. Water is absorbed in the large intestine (**4**) where faeces are formed as the final digestive stage.

The small intestine is lined with tiny, finger-like projections called villi which increase its surface area for absorption of food to about 350 square yards. Here arteries, veins and lymph vessels (which carry fat around the body for release into the blood stream) carry off digested products. All that is left is a watery mix of fibrous waste, cellulose, salts and other products and this passes into the large intestine. About two-thirds of this is absorbed in the form of water. The rest builds up and passes out of the body as faeces.

WHERE FOOD IS DIGESTED

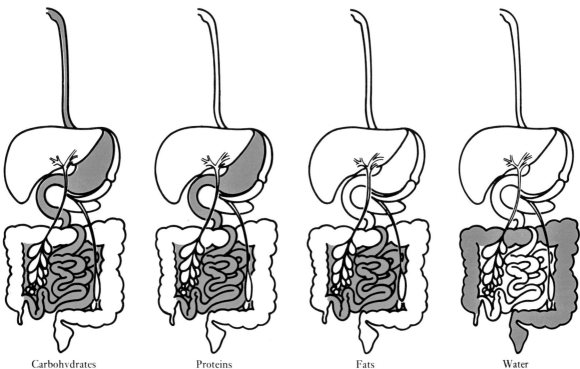

| Carbohydrates | Proteins | Fats | Water |

Although no single type of food is digested solely in one part of the system, there is a general pattern. Carbohydrates are the first to be acted on – in the mouth, oesophagus and stomach, the process finishing in the small intestine. Proteins are 'begun' in the stomach but mostly handled in the small intestine. Fats are actually dealt with in the small intestine. Finally, water is absorbed in the large intestine.

Digestion is a complex process which efficiently copes with all the different foods you eat and drink by extracting what is needed and dumping the rest. How long the process takes depends on what you eat, how much, and your health, but on average it takes about fifteen hours for food to go through the system.

BLOOD CIRCULATION

Your circulation system combines a delivery service with a waste disposal system, using blood as the transporter. It is a complex but highly efficient way for the body to feed itself with the chemicals and nutrients it needs for fuel and repair and to rid itself of the waste products created in the process of maintaining life.

How does it work? The powerhouse of circulation is the heart whose regular muscular contractions (about seventy a minute) maintain the flow of blood round the body.

The heart is two linked muscular pumps each consisting of an atrium which holds blood and a ventricle which pumps it.

The left side of the heart receives freshly oxygenated blood via the pulmonary veins from the lungs and stores it in the left atrium. This contracts to send the blood flowing into the left ventricle, which in turn pumps it out into the body through the arteries, starting with the largest of all, the aorta.

The blood reaches the end of its outward journey at the capillaries, minute vessels whose walls, only one cell thick, allow the passage of oxygen out from the blood to the cells and then take in carbon dioxide and other waste products.

The de-oxygenated blood travels up the capillaries into the veins which conduct it back to the right side of the heart. The right atrium receives it, releases it into the right ventricle which pumps it through the pulmonary artery to the lungs. There the carbon dioxide is expelled from the body as you breathe out. You then breathe in fresh oxygen and the whole process starts again.

In practice the right and left sides of the heart work together so that the atria and ventricles relax and contract at the same time, maintaining a balanced flow of blood round the body.

There is a difference between the two sides. The left side, because it does the heavy work of pumping the blood out through the arteries, is bigger. That is why your heart appears to beat on the left side of your chest even though it is centrally placed in the body.

Like all pumps the heart relies on valves to ensure that the blood only flows one way. The main ones lie between the left atrium and left ventricle (the mitral valve) and the right atrium and right ventricle (the tricuspid valve).

The circulatory system allows the blood to do its complex work all over the body – picking up nutrients from the intestines, transporting waste material, maintaining body temperature, regulating the water content of tissue cells and carrying the antibodies that fight infection. Little wonder then that diseases of the heart and arteries are so serious, and so often fatal.

THE PRINCIPAL ARTERIES AND VEINS

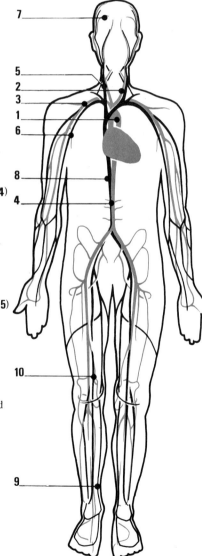

Arteries take fresh blood from the heart. The Aorta (**1**) leads from the left ventricle and is the most important. The carotid arteries (**2**) ascend the neck taking blood to the brain. The sub-clavian arteries (**3**) take blood into the arms and are used for pulse readings. The aorta leads to the abdominal aorta (**4**) serving the kidneys, intestine and liver. The femoral arteries take blood to the legs.
Veins transport blood back to the heart and lungs for re-oxygenation. The familiar jugular (**5**) vein lies behind and below the ear – and has a 'twin' inside the neck which you cannot feel. Brachial veins (**6**) receive blood from head, upper limbs and chest; blood drains from the head via the venous sinuses (**7**). The inferior vena cava (**8**) in the abdomen is a vital 'clearing' vein, back to the heart and the saphenous (**9**) and femoral (**10**) veins bring blood from the lower limbs.

34

A DOUBLE SYSTEM

Two of the most common checks that doctors make on us relate to blood and circulation – blood pressure and pulse rate.

YOUR BLOOD PRESSURE

This is the pressure that has to be applied to an artery to stop the pulse beyond the point of pressure. It is normally taken with an instrument called a sphygmomanometer – the familiar inflatable rubber bag that is strapped to your upper arm. It has two tubes leading out of it, one to a pressure gauge and the other to a hand pump. The bag is pumped up to restrict the flow of blood in the artery and the pressure is read when the pulse at the wrist or elbow disappears. Unusually high blood pressure may indicate disease of the arteries or kidneys, or stress.

YOUR PULSE

This is a useful quick check of the state of both your heart's action and your arteries.

Every time your heart beats and drives blood into the aorta, a fluid muscular wave runs down the arteries and they swell momentarily. You can feel it where an artery is near the surface of the body – notably an inch or so above the inside of the wrist.

The pulse beats in rhythm with the heart – about seventy times a minute – though it is faster in childhood and slower in old age. Your pulse will be faster too if you have a fever or have exerted yourself.

HOW TO TAKE YOUR PULSE

You need a clock or watch with a second hand in view. If you have a watch wear it on your left wrist and place the tips of the left-hand fingers at the base of the right-hand thumb. You will quickly find the pulse. Count the beats for fifteen seconds and multiply by four for your pulse rate per minute.

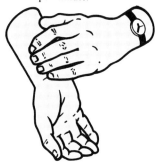

THE HEART

Aorta

Pulmonary veins

Pulmonary artery

Atrium left

Atrium right

Tricuspid valve

Mitral valve

Ventricle left

Ventricle right

WHAT IS BLOOD?

Blood is made up of . . .

Plasma This is about 90 per cent water and 8 per cent soluble proteins. The rest contains glucose, amino acids, fats, vitamins, hormones, urea, salts.

Red cells These transport the gases round the body. They contain haemoglobin which gives blood its red colour.

White cells These help to protect the body from infection by attacking and destroying bacteria.

Platelets Produced by special cells in the bone marrow. When you cut yourself they release a chemical which causes blood to clot.

BLOOD CELLS

 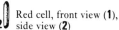

Red cell, front view (**1**), side view (**2**)

One of the many kinds of white cell

Platelets

THE URINARY SYSTEM

As your body processes the food you eat and air you breathe so it produces waste products, just like any manufacturer. It has four ways of getting rid of the waste – by breathing out carbon dioxide; excreting water, salts and urea (an end product of protein) through the skin; the excretion of bile salts, cellulose and other fibrous waste in the faeces; and in urine.

The urinary system is the most important of these four waste disposal methods and its key organs are the two kidneys. Each is 4 inches long, $2\frac{1}{2}$ inches wide and $1\frac{1}{2}$ inches thick. What they do is separate water and soluble solids from the blood as it is pumped under great pressure through them from the renal artery. About 2500 pints of blood are pumped through each day so, considering their small size, it is easy to imagine the pressure under which they work.

Each one is a collection of tiny filtration units shaped like cups and called nephrons. When blood enters one of these it passes into a tiny knot of capillaries whose walls allow waste products to pass out. This waste is directed from each

nephron to a central collecting point in the kidney called the renal pelvis.

Here the waste gathers as urine and passes down a 10-inch tube (the ureter) to the bladder where up to a pint can be stored until it is passed through the urethra and out of the body. The urethra is the only part of the urinary system that varies between men and women in an important way. Because it passes all the way down the penis it is longer in men – about 8 inches compared to only $1\frac{1}{2}$ inches long in women. For men too it serves a double function as it is also the passage down which their sperm travels in an ejaculation.

In practice, most of what passes through the kidneys is re-absorbed into the body, for once blood from the renal artery has been filtered it passes out again via the renal vein. Kidney failure can be fatal as too much waste goes back into the body – this can happen if there is chronic infection, diabetes or high blood pressure, and artificial kidney machines may then have to be used.

HOW KIDNEYS WORK

The kidneys clean blood that comes in through the renal arteries. Their filtration units are the minute nephrons which extract waste as urine, passing it into a collecting point, the renal pelvis, then down the ureters to the bladder. Muscles at the sphincter release urine into the urethra as the bladder fills, passing it out of the body. Meanwhile the purified blood passes back into circulation through the renal veins.

WHAT IS URINE

Urine is 96 per cent water, the rest being soluble solids. These include urea (a waste product formed by the liver), minerals like potassium, calcium, magnesium, phosphates and sulphates, uric acid, a little ammonia (which gives it its main smell) and pigments (derived from the blood).

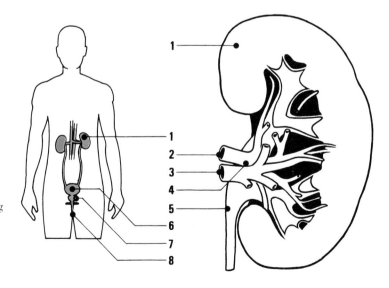

MALE URINARY SYSTEM
1 The kidneys and their location in the body
2 Renal artery
3 Renal vein
4 Renal pelvis
5 Ureter
6 Bladder
7 Sphincter
8 Urethra

THE LIVER

Your liver is your body's main chemical processing plant, operating day and night to perform a bewildering variety of processes on which life and health depend, as the list below suggests.

The liver weighs about 3 pounds; it is the biggest gland in the body and is situated beneath the ribs on the upper right-hand side of the abdomen. It uses enzymes to process the fats, amino acids and glucose that are fed into it by a continual 'washing' of blood – at the rate of about $2\frac{1}{2}$ pints a minute. The blood is fed into the liver from two sources: the hepatic artery supplies it with freshly oxygenated blood from the heart, while the hepatic portal vein brings blood from the digestive organs with nutrients ready for processing and absorption into the body.

The basic units of the liver are the hepatic cells, themselves grouped into between 50,000 and 100,000 lobules. Each of these is infiltrated with arterial and portal blood vessels as well as ducts for bile.

A two-way traffic takes place as the hepatic cells take oxygen and nutrients from the arterial and portal vessels and secrete into the blood glucose, vitamins, proteins, fats and other compounds needed by the millions of different cells of the body. A maze of vessels drains blood from the lobules to the hepatic vein which carries it out of the liver after it has been processed.

The bile produced by the hepatic cells is transported to the gall bladder which feeds it, as it is needed, through the bile ducts, to the intestine. One of the important protections the liver gives us lies in its ability to detoxify poisonous material that we may try to digest. Alcohol is a good example, for without the intercession of the liver it would accumulate in the blood in lethal concentrations.

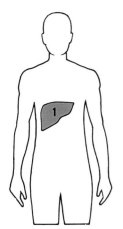

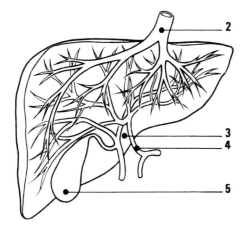

THE LIVER'S CAPACITY FOR RENEWAL

Unlike the other glands of the body the liver can reconstitute itself if it is damaged in any way or a part removed. It can, in fact, function effectively if only one-fifth of its tissue remains intact – one reason why disease of the liver may go unnoticed until it is well advanced.

THE LIVER
1 The liver and its location in the body
2 Hepatic vein
3 Portal vein
4 Hepatic artery
5 Gall bladder

FUNCTIONS OF THE LIVER

Here are some important functions of the liver:
– stores carbohydrates in the form of glycogen as an energy reserve
– makes fibrinogen, the substance needed for blood clotting
– recovers iron from red blood corpuscles
– stores iron, especially in the embryo baby
– stores Vitamin B12, needed by adults for the proper functioning of bone marrow
– gives the body warmth from the heat released by its many chemical processes
– makes the bile, the solution of organic compounds which partially aid digestion and helps get rid of waste products
– forms Vitamin A (retinol) needed for healthy skin and night vision
– processes and stores fats
– gets rid of the waste product ammonia in urea, which is sent to the kidneys
– provides fuel for muscles
– stores copper
– removes poisons
– contains salts which emulsify fats

37

THE REPRODUCTIVE SYSTEM

Like many of the other body systems the reproductive system has several roles, for in addition to reproduction it is also involved in releasing the hormones which trigger off puberty in boys and girls. This results in the development of the secondary sexual characteristics, for example the growth of facial hair and the deepening of the voice in boys and the development of breasts and the start of ovulation in girls. However, unlike the other systems, the reproductive system is unusually wasteful of its resources. Millions of male sperm and hundreds of female eggs are produced and yet, out of these, only a very few will actually fulfil their function, fuse and finally produce another human being.

Sexual intercourse between the two sexes occurs when the penis enters the vagina and ejaculates sperm with considerable force so that it comes as near to the cervix as possible.

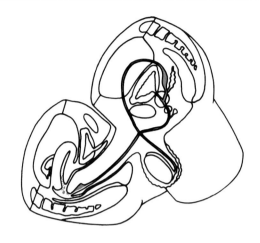

SPERM ROUTE
After ejaculation sperm swim up the vagina, through the womb and into the fallopian tube. The sperm have a twelve-hour life. It can take this long for one sperm to penetrate a female egg.

THE MALE REPRODUCTIVE ORGANS

A man has two external organs – the penis and two testes (held in the scrotum). But, as the drawing shows, there is more to it than that.

The job of each testis is to produce spermatozoa, which fertilise the female egg. Each testis is $1\frac{1}{2}$–2 inches long and sperm are formed from puberty onwards in thin tubes inside them. Between the tubes are cells which make the male hormone testosterone.

Ducts in each testis carry the sperm to its epididymis, an oblong tube at the top of each testis in which the sperm develop and mature. They mature over about three weeks and are carried up to the vas deferens, one for each testis, and deposited in the seminal vesicle, a sac at the juncture of the vas deferens and the urethra. Here the sperm combine with seminal fluid made by both the seminal vesicles and the prostate gland, a sac at the juncture of the vas deferens and the urethra.

The sperm themselves are minute – it would take about a thousand of them to cover the full stop at the end of this sentence. Before the sperm can leave the body they must travel down the urethra (valves leading to the bladder prevent the mixing of urine and sperm) and then to the penis.

The penis' ability to enlarge and grow erect depends on three columns of spongy tissue which ran down its length. Sexual arousal makes these fill with blood whose outflow from the penis is restricted so that it swells and grows stiff. In this state it can enter a woman's body and release sperm at the end of her vagina.

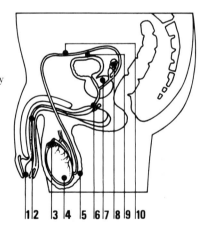

1 Penis
2 Spongy tissues
3 Epididymis
4 Testis
5 Scrotum
6 Urethra   ,
7 Prostate gland
8 Seminal vesicle
9 Bladder
10 Vas deferens

THE AVERAGE MENSTRUAL CYCLE

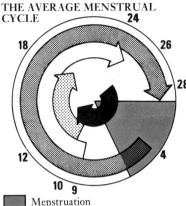

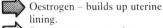
Menstruation

Oestrogen – builds up uterine lining.

Progesterone – completes creation of uterine lining.

FSH (Follicle Stimulating Hormone) – stimulates the follicle.

LH (Luteinising Hormone) – causes ovulation.

The numbers refer to days in the menstrual cycle.

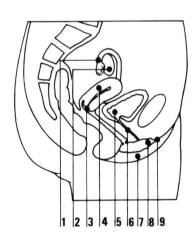

```
1  2  3  4  5  6  7  8  9
```

1 Fallopian tube
2 Ovary
3 Cervix
4 Uterus
5 Bladder
6 Urethra
7 Labia majora
8 Labia minora
9 Clitoris

OVULATION

A woman's menstrual cycle usually runs over about twenty-eight days. At the beginning of the month the hypothalamus at the base of the brain releases a hormone which stimulates the ovary follicles to grow. One follicle will grow faster than the rest and in the second week a second hormone stimulates it to burst and release an egg.

As ovulation takes place the broken follicle fills with blood and a yellow fatty material and the womb lining thickens with extra layers of tissue containing blood vessels and glands.

The egg, meanwhile, makes its way into the fallopian tube where, should sperm be present, fertilisation may take place. If it doesn't then the egg will die about two days later. The lining of the womb starts to break down, as does the substance in the follicle. In about the fourth week blood and pieces of tissue and the unwanted egg flow out of the womb, into the vagina and the menstrual flow occurs.

THE FEMALE REPRODUCTIVE ORGANS

A woman's reproductive organs are essentially internal.

There are four of them – the ovaries, the fallopian tubes, the uterus and the vagina. The two ovaries are the size of plums and situated just above the uterus on either side of it. Every woman is born with 50,000 or so follicles in her ovaries, each containing one egg, which ripen and are released from puberty at about eleven years of age to the menopause in her late forties when menstruation ceases and her reproductive life is over.

The fallopian tubes link the ovaries and uterus (the womb) and it is here that fertilisation takes place. Each tube is about 4 inches long.

The uterus is pear-shaped and rather smaller than a fist. Its walls are muscular to give the force necessary for birth, and are lined with mucous membrane (endometrium), which has the role of nurturing any eggs that are fertilised. The uterus is linked to the vagina by the cervix. The vagina receives the penis during intercourse and allows the passage of sperm into the uterus and fallopian tubes. Normally the vagina is

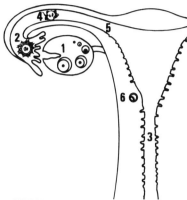

FERTILIZATION
The order of events would be:
1 Ovulation
2 Ovum in Fallopian tube
3 Entry of sperm in vagina, uterus, fallopian tube
4 Fertilization of ovum
5 Ovum travels down Fallopian Tube
6 Ovum implanted in lining of Uterus (the endometrium).

quite narrow, its walls of folded skin lying close together. In intercourse they become moist and stretch easily, to facilitate the entry of the penis.

The cervix is full of thick mucus which prevents the passage upwards of small particles – but during ovulation this becomes thin and watery so that sperm may successfully pass through it into the uterus.

At the vaginal opening are protective folds of tissue – the labia majora and minora – and the clitoris, a small bud-shaped organ which is sensitive to sexual arousal – and may trigger it off. Here too is the exit of the urethra, the urinary passage from the bladder.

THE NERVOUS SYSTEM

Your body uses its nervous system to tell itself what responses to make at any particular moment in every part of itself to maintain life and health. It continually monitors information from both outside and inside the body. This is fed into the brain and endocrine systems and they in turn tell the body how to react.

If you, for example, accidentally pick up a pan with a burning hot handle your nervous system will trigger a reflex action in the muscles of your arm and hand and cause you to drop it. However, you will override this instruction without seeming to think about it if there's a baby at your feet.

The central nervous system which regulates such complex responses is controlled by the brain which weighs about 3 pounds (or 2 per cent of your body weight) and is cushioned in a watery fluid protected by the skull. Its functions are so important that it absorbs one-fifth of the oxygen and blood the body needs.

Over 30,000 million nerve units process most of the information which enables you to live and also

THE NERVOUS SYSTEM

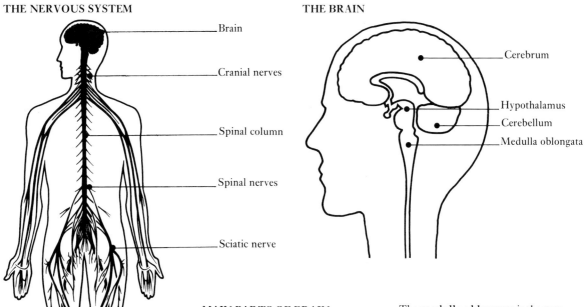

- Brain
- Cranial nerves
- Spinal column
- Spinal nerves
- Sciatic nerve

THE BRAIN

- Cerebrum
- Hypothalamus
- Cerebellum
- Medulla oblongata

MAIN PARTS OF BRAIN
The main part of the brain is the **cerebrum** occupying a bigger portion of the brain than in any other warm-blooded mammal and giving man his unique mental characteristics.

It is divided into two parts. The left side, regulating the right-hand side of the body, controls abilities like writing, talking and mathematics. The right side controls the left-hand side of the body and non-verbal abilities – making spatial judgements, artistic ability, appreciation of music.

The **medulla oblongata** is the stem connecting the brain with the spinal column and houses the autonomic nervous system, which maintains day-to-day basics like breathing and digestion.

The **cerebellum** is under the back of the brain where it joins the stem and is responsible for balance and complex muscular control.

The **hypothalamus** is a prune-sized organ in the centre of the brain richly supplied with blood. It is a sort of central switchboard through which many nerve impulses are fed.

gives you senses and feelings. You may think you hear, see or smell directly with your ears, eyes and nose but the information giving you these senses is processed and interpreted in the brain.

The telephone systems of the body are the nerves which connect the brain with the rest of the body. They range in size from the microscopic to one which is the thickness of a pencil (the sciatic nerve in the thigh). They use the spinal cord as a main highway branching off to all parts of the body. Impulses are sent back and forth by electro-chemical reactions and at speeds of up to 300 feet a second.

Twelve pairs of cranial nerves from the underside of the brain connect with the main organs of the head, chest and abdomen controlling information about smell, sight and hearing.

The thirty-one pairs of spinal nerves spread across the body to the hands and feet. Some you are aware of – particularly those concerned with touch – but many may act swiftly to save your life without you even realising it.

FLIGHT OR FIGHT

The most dramatic example of how quick and effective the nerves can be is when the sympathetic nervous system goes into action. This is the defence mechanism which activates the body if it is faced with danger. Nerves running to the internal organs and tissues will do several things at once to prepare the body for action or flight.

Once the danger is past, the body automatically goes into reverse so that everything can revert smoothly to normal.

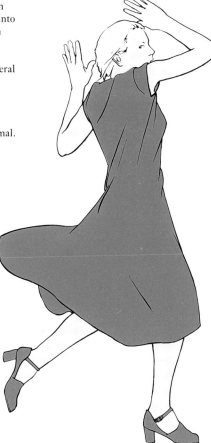

Eyes: pupils dilate so that more light can enter and vision is sharper.

Heart rate increases and blood flows faster to allow the body to act quickly

Lungs relax so that more air can enter

Liver pushes more glucose into the body for extra energy

Blood vessels become wider, making it possible to push more oxygen to the muscles, while the vessels feeding less important areas like the skin contract (which is why you go white with fear)

SYSTEMS FOR LIFE AND CHANGE

The constant chemical changes in the body's tissues, and the physical and chemical processes which maintain life, are called metabolism.

What is most interesting about metabolism is the way in which it is regulated internally so that the hundreds of thousands of processes involved in your body are harmonised and in balance.

The central organ concerned is your liver (see page 37) with various hormonal glands (see opposite) regulating many specialised processes such as the chemistry of growth, sex, digestion, and reactions to danger.

Our metabolic needs – the energy we require to maintain body functions – vary with both our age and sex, **and** with the particular activity we are doing.

The simplest way to express this is the basal metabolic rate (BMR) – the amount of energy, measured in calories or joules **in relation to our body weight,** we need to maintain the basics like heartbeat, warmth, respiration **while at rest.**

Because babies and children are growing their metabolic rate is faster than adults although the total amount of calories they consume is normally less. Among adults the average man's BMR is faster than a woman's since it is proportional to the amount of muscle each has. Old people, who are less active, have a lower BMR.

What the liver does is to filter amino acids and carbohydrates out of the blood after it has picked up nutrients from the digestive organs. The liver controls the supply of nutrients like glycogen and several vitamins, storing and releasing them as our metabolic needs for them vary.

Not only do the metabolic processes take care of the whole body – they also ensure that the most important parts of it are protected when there is a shortage. So, for example, the brain has the first call on glucose in the body – other organs using other fuels if there is a shortage. And when food is very short the metabolic rate falls so that the body consumes less to maintain life.

HOW YOUR ENERGY NEEDS CHANGE . . .

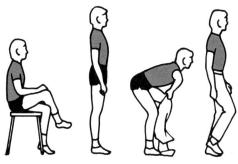

● One calorie burned each minute

Figures for an average twenty-five-year-old 65-kg man – but the relative differences are the same for most people.

EVERYDAY ACTIVITIES
-)● Sitting
-)● Standing
-)●●● Washing, dressing
- ●●● Walking slowly
- ●●●●● Walking moderately quickly
- ●●●●●●●●● Walking up and down stairs

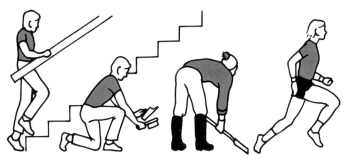

WORK AND RECREATION

)●●)●● ⎰ Most domestic work
Golf
Lorry driving
Light industrial and assembly work
⎱ Carpentry, bricklaying

)●●●●●●● ⎰ Gardening
Tennis, dancing
Cycling to 20 km per hour
Digging, shovelling
⎱ Agricultural work

)●●●●●●● ⎰ Coal mining, steel furnace work
and over Squash, cross country running
⎱ Football, swimming (crawl)

SO WHAT CONTROLS YOUR BODY?

The Endocrine System

Most of us think we control our own bodies. After all, we decide when to work, when to have a bath, when to eat. But this is only true up to a point. What is it that decides when you are so tired that you fall asleep at work? Or that water is too hot to have a bath in? Or that some of what you eat is not worth absorbing into the body?

The fact is that the constant chemical and physical changes within the body are so complex that it would be impossible to control them consciously. If we tried to the body would break down very quickly.

Two interrelated systems control these body processes. The endocrine and the central nervous systems.

The keys to the endocrine system are the hormones – chemical messengers whose job is to regulate processes of the body so that an internal balance is maintained. They are released mainly into the bloodstream from different glands spread through the body, each of whose function is different but vitally important.

HOW THE ENDOCRINE SYSTEM RESPONDS

When we run, or do heavy work in the garden, we become conscious of a host of body changes as our systems respond to the new demands put on them: we may sweat, pant, grow tired, start feeling hungry. Such vigorous activity increases our metabolic rate and we burn the fuel absorbed from our food faster. For this reason activity may help keep us slim. But what makes us put on weight is not inactivity, but too much food. The body takes advantage of a good surplus by converting some of the excess into fat which is stored in the adipose tissue. Neither the metabolic process nor the endocrine system has a built-in 'slimming control' and that is therefore something we have to consciously provide ourselves, except that those with a high metabolic rate have far fewer slimming problems.

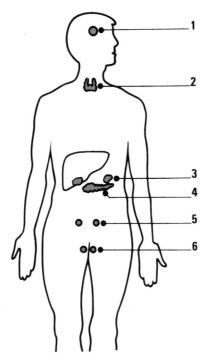

THE HORMONAL GLANDS

1 THE PITUITARY GLAND

This gland – the size of a pea – hangs from the base of the brain in a protective hollow in the skull. Its position indicates its great importance.

It controls growth, stimulates the contractions in the uterus to make normal birth possible and controls the action of the blood vessels. It also controls several other hormonal glands and triggers the onset of adolescence and maturity.

2 THE THYROID GLAND

Situated in front of the neck below the adam's apple, it controls the speed with which the body's cells turn food into energy.

If it is over-active (which may occur under stress) the body burns food very fast yet remains thin; if it is under-active then lethargy and obesity set in. Its main job is to regulate the body's nutritional needs.

3 ADRENAL GLANDS

The core of these two glands produces adrenalin, the hormone which triggers off a whole series of body reactions needed to make it act swiftly when faced by stress and danger.

Their outside layer regulates the processing of proteins, fats and carbo-hydrates and maintains the body's mineral and water balance. It also produces some sex hormones.

4 THE PANCREAS

Its job is to release into the small intestine enzymes which aid digestion. It produces two hormones which control the level of sugar in the blood – insulin which reduces it and glucagon which increases it.

5 THE OVARIES AND

6 TESTICLES

These pairs of glands in women and men play a key part in reproduction, releasing eggs and sperm and maintaining fertility. Also, during adolescence they respond to a signal from the pituitary gland to release hormones (oestrogen for women, testosterone for men) which give women and men their secondary sexual characteristics.

THE FOOD YOUR BODY NEEDS

Most people eat food from custom and habit with little real knowledge of what it does for their bodies. As most of us in the Western world have more than enough food to survive, we are rarely forced to think of our diet. Indeed most of us only worry about food when we eat too much. However, there is a difference between simply surviving and being really healthy. The fact is that despite a plentiful food supply there is growing evidence that many hundreds of thousands of people suffer from an unbalanced diet whose effects are serious in the long term but may be hard to detect from day to day. We have already seen (pages 16–17) how nutrient deficiencies can affect the health. This

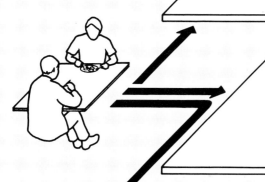

YOU NEED FOOD FOR THREE REASONS:

FUEL PROVIDERS

To provide the **fuel** that creates the energy needed to stay alive, work and play. Energy comes from starch and sugar (the carbohydrates), fats and to a small extent from protein. Starch comes from cereals, seeds and root vegetables, and foods made from them. Sugar (proper name sucrose) is made

RAW MATERIAL SUPPLIERS

To supply the raw materials from which your body takes what it needs to build and repair itself. These are the foods which give the body the materials – particularly proteins – it needs to rebuild parts that get used up or deteriorate in the course of living. Protein is part of every one of the millions of cells

VITAL CHEMICALS

To make available the chemicals that are the basis of the reactions and processes which make your body's self-maintenance possible.
The body also needs a number of chemicals and minerals to aid its chemical processes and help the work that the energy and material foods do. Carbohydrates cannot be converted into energy

chapter shows what contribution different foods make to health so that you can find out what you gain by adding the right foods to your diet. It is important to realise that there is no such thing as a 'perfect' diet. Even if nutritionists could provide accurate quantities of what **you** should eat (which will be different from someone else and also vary from time to time) it would be technically impossible for the average person to measure out the right quantities. In practice your body has mechanisms which extract the right nutrients at the right time **provided** it is given them in your diet. So your task is to get into eating habits that achieve this. These pages will help you do so.

from sugar beet, cane or maple and is likely to be found in most sweet foods and in drinks like beer, sherry and cider. A third supplier of energy is fat – animal and vegetable. Sources include butter, oils, milk, cereal, meat and nuts. Protein and alcohol also provide fuel for the body, though to a lesser extent.

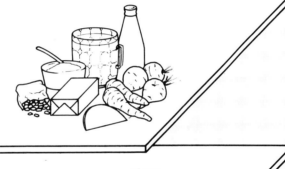

from which the body is built – it forms our building blocks. No food is pure protein, but some are more protein-rich than others. These include fish, meat, poultry, cheese, milk and yogurt, nuts, beans and cereals. Bread is also important as a protein provider because it is a significant part of Western diet.

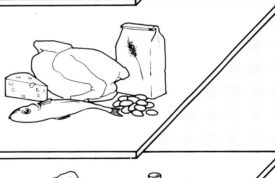

without Vitamin B1. Most vitamins cannot be made by the body, so they **must** be supplied by food. Minerals like calcium (for bones and teeth) and iron (for healthy blood) are needed too, usually in tiny amounts. While the average diet provides most of these chemicals it may also give you too much carbohydrate or too little of some of the vitamins and minerals.

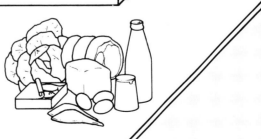

CARBOHYDRATES

THE ENERGY PROVIDERS

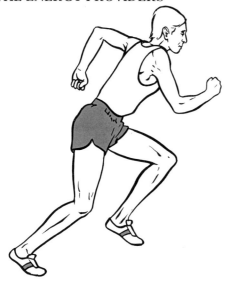

Carbohydrate is the great energy provider without which most diets – in both East and West – would look very bare indeed. This is because foods rich in carbohydrate, such as potatoes, rice and flour, tend to be bulky, forming the main component of most normal diets.

More and more people are now aware of the dangers of being overweight and because of this carbohydrates have wrongly got a bad name.

The problem is that if they are taken in excess, especially in a refined form, then, like sugar, they are stored in the body as fat. Because of this real danger many popular slimming diets give the impression that all that carbohydrate-rich foods provide are calories, and this is certainly not the

Carbohydrates come in several forms – the three major categories being starches, cellulose and sugars.

STARCH

Starch is the major solid ingredient of cereals, root vegetables and pulses. It is formed from many different glucose units and supplies most of the energy used by people in their diet.

In Britain, starch provides the bulk of the carbohydrates we normally consume – of the rest most comes from sucrose and the remainder from lactose.

Because they are insoluble in water most starches are hard to digest raw, which is why we normally cook high-starch foods like potatoes and flour. Cooking makes the starch granules swell and gelatinise so they can be more easily digested.

CELLULOSE AND RELATED MATERIALS

This kind of carbohydrate is indigestible for man. However, it is very valuable as fibre or roughage which helps the formation of faeces and the passage of waste products through the intestines. Research suggests that such fibre is important in preventing cancer of the colon. You can increase the fibre in your diet by switching from white bread, soft drinks and products made with white flour to whole grain cereals, fresh fruit and vegetables.

SUGARS

There are five main types of sugars.

Glucose: This is found in some fruit and plant juices and is the sugar into which most carbohydrates are converted by digestion.

Fructose – Found in some fruit and vegetables, but most familiarly in honey. It is very sweet – much more so than refined white sugar.

Sucrose This is a combination of glucose and fructose and is what most people mean by 'sugar'. It is found in small quantities in sugar cane, sugar beet and in most fruits and root vegetables, especially carrots.

Maltose – This is formed when starch is broken down as in the course of digestion or in the production of malt beer.

Lactose – This is only found in milk and milk products and recent research shows that it can only be dealt with by the body if the enzyme lactase is present. Sugars are used mainly as sweeteners, energy providers and as preservatives in jam making, canning, bottling and freezing. Refined white sugar provides what some nutritionists call 'empty' calories – energy without nutrients. Many brown sugars too often contain only colouring and are mainly sucrose. Sugar is responsible for the high incidence of dental caries (cavities) because it provides the right fuel in which the bacteria causing tooth decay can thrive.

case. As the table of foods providing carbohydrates suggests, many of them are also providers of vitamins, proteins, fibre and minerals, all of which are vital to good health. So if you are suddenly going to cut back on carbohydrates you must make sure these other nutrients are going to be provided from elsewhere; otherwise your health will be at risk. It is worth stressing that it is hard to provide the energy that the body needs with an acceptable diet unless you have some carbohydrate foods in it. However, as sugar and sugar-rich foods tend to provide only empty calories, that is one source of carbohydrates that you can safely cut back on. Carbohydrate is an important part of the diet because it can't be stored in the body as minerals can (except in the form of fat and, in relatively small quantities, in the form of glycogen). Carbohydrates, which are made up of carbon, hydrogen and oxygen, are relatively easily digested by the body, as you would expect of the food that provides us with fuel. However, recent research has shown that one of the sugars, lactose, which is found in milk, requires the presence of an enzyme called lactase before it can be absorbed by the body. Most Europeans have enough lactase in their intestine to cope with the lactose they consume, but some coloured populations, particularly those of African origin, along with most Chinese, do not have sufficient lactase to handle lactose.

WHERE DO WE GET CARBOHYDRATES FROM?

Starch is the main carbohydrate source – most of it coming from potato and flour-based products, as the table below shows. Perhaps surprisingly, sugar – also an important source of carbohydrate – would not occur naturally in the diet (except for that in fruit and milk) were it not used as a sweetener and preservative in foods like tinned fruit and jams.

On pages 114–115 we look in more detail at how to approach slimming but we should always remember with carbohydrates that much of your intake **is** likely to be in the form of refined sugar (sucrose) – whether directly spooned or indirectly as part of a processed food. The average consumption of sugar is now 2 pounds per person per week. It makes sense therefore, if you want to cut back on calories, to start by reducing your consumption of these 'empty' calorie providers.

CARBOHYDRATE CONTENT OF SOME FOODS

SUGAR FOODS	% of carbo-hydrate	CEREALS	% of carbo-hydrate	FRUIT	% of carbo-hydrate	VEGETABLES	% of carbo-hydrate	ANIMAL PRODUCE	% of carbo-hydrate
food		food		food		food		food	
sugar	100	rice (polished, uncooked)	87	raisins	64	potatoes	21	milk (fresh whole)	5
syrup	79	white flour	80	dates	64	baked beans in tomato sauce	10	condensed milk (whole sweetened)	56
jam	69	wholemeal flour	73	bananas	19	parsnips	11	evaporated milk	
		oatmeal (raw)	73	grapes	15	cabbage (winter, raw)	3	(whole unsweetened)	11
		white bread	54	apples (whole)	9	runner beans	4	liver (lamb's)	16
		wholemeal bread	47	pears	8	peas (frozen)	7	most other meats	
						spinach	1	and fish	0

FATS

THE ENERGY CONSERVERS

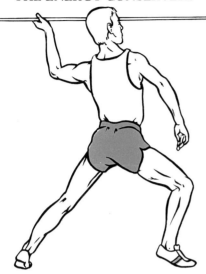

Fats play a far bigger all-round role in diet and enjoyment of food than most people realise. They have four important functions:

PROVIDING ENERGY

Fats are the most concentrated form of energy in foods – having twice as much per gramme as carbohydrates or proteins. So they can give you energy in a much more concentrated way than bulky carbohydrates. The body, ever efficient, prefers to store its energy in the form of fat, which is why excess carbohydrate is turned into fat before being stored, where it has the additional role of insulating the body.

MAKING FOOD PALATABLE

Fat's ability to make food more palatable is acknowledged in many of the combinations that make up popular everyday foods and dishes. Bread and butter is the classic example but there

THE DIFFERENT TYPES OF FAT

What is fat? . . . and is it dangerous? There are many types of fat, all of them combinations of carbon, hydrogen and oxygen. From a health point of view it is useful to understand the difference between **saturated** and **polyunsaturated** fats. This is because saturated fats may increase the level of one potentially dangerous fat – cholesterol – in our blood if we consume too much of them. Unsaturated fats have fewer hydrogen molecules than saturated fats but you don't need to be a scientist to tell the difference. Saturated fats like butter and lard are solid at room temperature while (with very few exceptions) unsaturated fats are liquid, like corn, soya and sunflower oils.

Where does cholesterol come into the picture? The body makes its own supply of cholesterol which it uses principally for the vital job of building brain tissue. It does not really need any more from outside but because our consumption of solid fats is so high (it has increased dramatically in the last century) it gets it. Nutritionists call this **dietary cholesterol**.

Cholesterol goes into the bloodstream and may start furring up the arteries, a condition called atherosclerosis. This is a condition common in old age but it seems that the wrong diet may create the condition earlier in life. As a result arteries may become blocked, causing coronary thrombosis or (if in the arteries of the brain) a stroke.

The cause of atherosclerosis is not fully understood but its association with the consumption of saturated fats is well enough established to make it advisable to consume polyunsaturated fats rather than saturated fats when possible. Use butter substitutes, and try to switch when possible from meat and eggs to cottage cheese, vegetables, nuts and wheatgerm. The reason why eggs should not be taken in excess is because although they are relatively low in fat as a whole, the yolk in its raw state is about 1.6 per cent cholesterol. So if you are a heavy egg eater cut down your consumption.

If you are planning to cut back on your fat intake you will find the table on this page very helpful (and see also pp.114–115: diets and slimming). It now seems sensible to reduce your intake of the saturated (usually animal) fats which are high in cholesterol and lower in the essential fatty acids.

are many others. Potatoes tend to be more attractive with a little butter or fat, while fish like cod and plaice (non-fatty fish) are usually cooked with a fatty sauce or in batter. (Fat fish like mackerel or herring do not need this addition to make them palatable.) Salads, too, are more appealing with an oily dressing.

CARRYING FAT – SOLUBLE VITAMINS
Four vitamins – A, D, E, and K – are normally taken into the body as part of fatty foods because they are soluble in fats.
Vitamin A is found in foods like cheese, liver, and fatty fish; D is found especially in fatty fish, while E is associated with vegetable oils, cereal products and eggs; K is widespread in vegetables and vegetable oils.

REMEMBER . . . the amount of food also affects your total fat intake. For example, because we consume large quantities of milk in Britain its importance as a source of fat is greater than is suggested by its position on the table.

SUPPLYING IMPORTANT NUTRIENTS
Edible fats also transport the three compounds which the body can't make for itself, linoleic acid, linolenic acid and arachidonic acid. These are now believed to be vital for growth, for helping the formation of the sex and adrenal hormones and possibly in the fat part of cell structure. But few of us need worry that we are deficient in any of these fatty acids since the amount we need is provided many times over in normal diets.

HOW FATTY ARE DAILY FOODS?

MEAT, FISH AND EGGS	avg % fat	VEGETABLES	avg % fat	CEREALS	avg % fat	DAIRY PRODUCE	avg % fat	FAT-CONTAINING PRODUCTS	avg % fat
eggs	11	peanuts	49	bread – wholemeal	3	butter	82	cooking oil	99.9
bacon – back	41	potatoes	trace	bread – white	2	cream	48	lard/dripping	99
beef – stewing steak	11			flour – white	1	cheese – cheddar	34	margarine	81
lamb – cutlets	36			oatmeal – raw	9	cheese – cottage	4	low-fat margarine	41
chicken	18					milk – whole fresh	3.8	ice cream – dairy	7
herring	19					milk – fresh skimmed	trace	ice cream – non dairy	8
fish – white (e.g. cod)	1								

49

PROTEINS

THE BODY BUILDERS

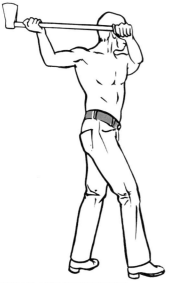

Proteins go to the heart of life itself because they are essential to the creation and maintenance of cells and the work they do.

Their importance in nutrition is unconsciously recognised by all of us because they normally make up such an important part of main meals. They are contained in the meat, fish, eggs, cheese, milk, peas, beans, nuts and cereals around which we build so many dishes.

WHAT ARE PROTEINS?

Proteins are made up of amino acids – chemical compounds combining nitrogen, carbon, hydrogen and oxygen. There are about twenty amino acids in the average Western diet, which combine to form thousands of different permutations. Eight of these amino acids are considered essential for adults. They cannot be made in the body, they must be provided in the diet. They are: isoleucine, leucine, lysine, methionine, phenylalanine, threonine, tryptophan and valine. A ninth, histidine, is essential for infants.

Most protein-providing foods lack at least one of these essential acids. Bread, for example, is short of lysine, and leafy vegetables are short of methionine. Though the body can store some foods, it is unable to store amino acids, so it cannot make proteins unless it has the right combination of amino acids with which to do so.

WHAT THEY DO

Proteins and the amino acids which form them are constantly needed for the rebuilding of cells since about 1 or 2 per cent of the body's tissue protein is being replaced every day. Different parts of the body require different amounts. Organs such as the heart, liver and kidneys, which are in constant active use, need more than do muscles and bones, whose protein turnover is slower.

Proteins also produce enzymes, which cause chemical reactions in the body necessary to maintain life. The enzymes in saliva, for instance, which are at the start of the digestive process, are made from proteins.

HOW MUCH PROTEIN DO WE NEED

For most people, eating a normal meat diet, there is no problem. The average male adult in Britain, for example, will consume about 90 g of protein a day – well in excess of the minimum. Nutritionists vary in their estimates of what we need but officially recommended intakes put the figure at 65 g a day for a sedentary man between the age of thirty-five and sixty-five years. Although, on average, most of us eat enough protein in the right combinations of amino acids there are some people who should be careful. These include babies at weaning, adolescents (who need protein for growth), convalescents (who need it for rebuilding), and nursing mothers (who need it to maintain the protein quality of their milk).

Vegetarians should also allow for protein needs. The new soya-derived texturised vegetable protein (TVP) caters especially for them. It is also a useful meat substitute for meat eaters – and well worth trying, especially as meat protein is becoming increasingly expensive for both the individual and the world as a whole.

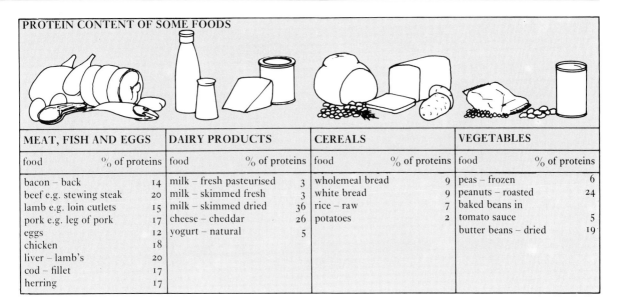

PROTEIN CONTENT OF SOME FOODS

MEAT, FISH AND EGGS		DAIRY PRODUCTS		CEREALS		VEGETABLES	
food	% of proteins	food	% of proteins	food	% of proteins	food	% of proteins
bacon – back	14	milk – fresh pasteurised	3	wholemeal bread	9	peas – frozen	6
beef e.g. stewing steak	20	milk – skimmed fresh	3	white bread	9	peanuts – roasted	24
lamb e.g. loin cutlets	15	milk – skimmed dried	36	rice – raw	7	baked beans in	
pork e.g. leg of pork	17	cheese – cheddar	26	potatoes	2	tomato sauce	5
eggs	12	yogurt – natural	5			butter beans – dried	19
chicken	18						
liver – lamb's	20						
cod – fillet	17						
herring	17						

WHERE DO WE GET PROTEINS

Only two foods provide, on their own, the perfect balance of amino acids – eggs and mother's milk. The first, eggs, cannot be eaten all the time and the latter we consume for only a short period in our lives. So, for good health, we should aim to eat a variety of protein foods simultaneously. Animal proteins generally provide a more balanced range of amino acids than vegetable sources, even though all protein is ultimately derived from plant material. This is because when animals eat plants they convert the proteins into combinations nearer to that required by humans.

This is one of the main reasons why vegetarians need to be more aware of what they are eating in protein terms than meat eaters – to make sure they get the full range necessary for health. In Britain about one-third of the protein in the average diet comes from that typical carbohydrate food – flour and its products. Although they have a relatively low protein content they form such a staple part of our diet that this content becomes significant in the total amount of what we eat. The best diets provide meals which give a variety of protein foods at the same time. Baked beans on toast, for example, is nicely balanced because while bread is low on lysine it is rich in methionine; the beans are low in methionine but rich in lysine. Eat them together and you'll have the right combination of amino acids with which to start the process of body building and repair.

BALANCED COMBINATIONS OF PROTEINS

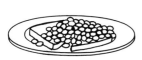

beans on toast

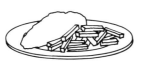

fish and chips

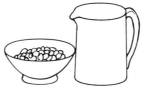

cereals and milk

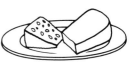

bread and cheese

VITAMINS

THE BODY BOOSTERS

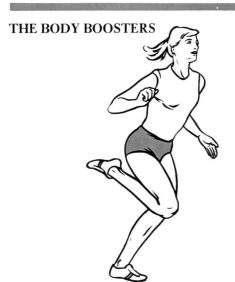

We need vitamins in only tiny amounts (less than 1 per cent of the diet) but they are vital to health and well being.

What they do principally is to help the body's metabolism, the process by which chemical changes occur which allow the body to renew itself. Extreme vitamin deficiency causes a wide range of disease of which scurvy, resulting from lack of Vitamin C, is perhaps the best known.

The wide availability of fresh citrus fruit, which provides Vitamin C, means that this is now very rare indeed. Other vitamin-deficiency diseases include osteomalacia (softening of bones) associated with a lack of Vitamin D plus a lack of sunshine; and an extreme form of anaemia resulting from a lack of Vitamin B12.

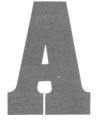 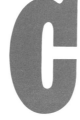 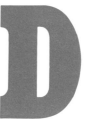

VITAMIN A
Chemical name: Retinol
It maintains the eyes' ability to adapt to the dark and keeps skin in good condition. A deficiency can damage the eyes and cause blindness, a common situation among children in many undeveloped countries where diet is unbalanced. Taken in excess it can accumulate in the liver and poison the body. Vitamin A is not widely distributed in food, the best sources being fish-liver oils followed by animal liver, kidney, daily produce and eggs. All margarine is required by law to contain the same amount of Vitamin A as best summer butter.

VITAMIN C
Chemical name: Ascorbic Acid
Vitamin C is needed to maintain healthy skin, ligaments and bones. It also promotes the absorption of iron. Daily requirements of Vitamin C may be higher than normal if you have a cold. Some scientists believe that massive doses of Vitamin C help colds but British government nutritionists are doubtful about this. It occurs in citrus fruits, blackcurrants, brussels sprouts and strawberries in relatively high concentrations. However, it is easily lost from fruit and vegetables, so the fresher they are the better.

VITAMIN D
Chemical name: Cholecalciferol
Promotes the absorption of calcium for the formation of normal bones. Infants and children who suffer from Vitamin D deficiency develop weak bones which are unable to support their weight and may be deformed as a result. For this reason in the United Kingdom Vitamin D preparations are given to pregnant women and to children. But too much can damage the kidneys. The sun creates Vitamin D by acting on a substance in the skin. Other sources include cod-liver oil, herring and eggs.

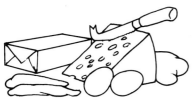 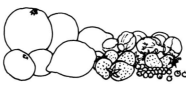 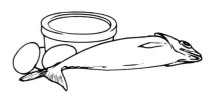

Some recent research by doctors specialising in nutrition suggests that big doses of certain vitamins (megavitamin therapy) may be a positive contribution to health, or solve specific conditions – but this is still a controversial field and needs medical supervision. It does nonetheless serve to underline the great importance to health of a part of our food which forms only a small proportion of the total we consume.

However, publicity about vitamins has the unfortunate result that they have come to be regarded as cure-alls, so that vitamin pills become part of some people's everyday diet. The fact is that a good all-round diet should provide all the vitamins you need naturally with no need for supplements. If you are going to supplement your diet with pills it **probably** won't do any harm because most vitamins are water-soluble, which means that excess amounts pass out of the body easily in urine. However, four vitamins (A, D, E and K) are fat-soluble and excessive intakes of these may be dangerous. The danger of supplements is that you may take too much of one of them. As you can't be certain what you are doing when you take vitamin supplements consult your doctor first. Don't be surprised if he says 'Go on to a good all-round diet', just as we do. There are thirteen vitamins known to be needed in our diet, of which eight are grouped under the umbrella of Vitamin B (the Vitamin B complex). Here are their names, functions, and the foods which are the commonest sources of them.

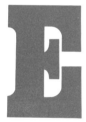

VITAMIN E
Chemical name: The group of substances labelled 'E' are tocopherols.
Its function is not yet fully understood. As most foods contain some Vitamin E and it is easily stored in the body, deficiency problems are unlikely. Especially good sources include eggs and oils derived from cereals such as wheat-germ oil, maize oil and cottonseed oil.

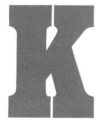

VITAMIN K
Chemical name: Phytomenadione
This is known as the anti-haemorrhagic vitamin because it is essential for the proper clotting of blood. It occurs in a wide range of foodstuffs of which green vegetables and fish-liver oils are perhaps the most important. Deficiency is very unlikely.

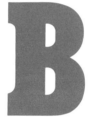

VITAMIN B COMPLEX
Includes: Thiamin, Riboflavin, Folic Acid and Biotin. Eight of the vitamins in this category are regarded as essential nutrients for humans, each one having a different function. They are all water-soluble and tend to occur in the same types of food so that a deficiency of one of them is unlikely, though in some extreme diets it does happen. Good sources for all of them are yeast extracts, whole grains, offal like liver and kidney, green vegetables, eggs and milk.

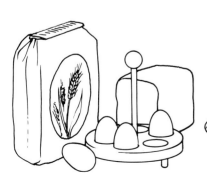

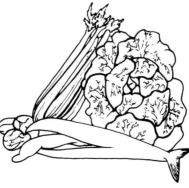

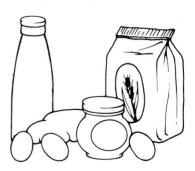

MINERALS

THE VITAL EXTRAS

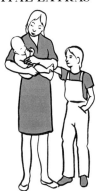

As nutritionists get to know more about the body's need for minerals, the clearer it becomes how much our health can depend on them. Because they often exist in such tiny amounts and their role is not always understood it is hard to measure how much of a particular mineral we need for health. It is only when there is a clear relationship between deficiency and ill health that nutritionists can say with confidence that we must have a given level of intake of a particular mineral. This occurs, for example, with iron (deficiency causes anaemia) and

Ca

CALCIUM
The average adult has about 42 oz (1200 g) of calcium in his body, 99 per cent of it in bones and teeth. Deficiency in it leads to the growth of stunted and malformed bones. This condition, known as rickets, can also occur if there is a shortage of Vitamin D in the diet because this is needed to help the body absorb calcium.

Naturally, the groups that need calcium most are growing children, pregnant women and nursing mothers. The recommended daily intake for the nine-to-fifteen age group is 700 mg, 600 mg for infants and 500 mg for adults. For a woman in the last three months of pregnancy it is 1200 mg a day. Although most calcium is needed for bones and teeth it is also needed to prevent osteoporosis (fragile bones) in old age and a lack of calcium can also result in tetany (muscular twitching). Best sources of it are milk, cheese, yogurt, sardines (in the bones) and white flour (to which it is added by government regulation).

Fe

IRON
This is the essential ingredient of haemoglobin, the pigment which gives blood its colour and acts as a carrier of oxygen in the blood from the lungs to the body tissues.

Over half of the body's 4 g of iron are used in this way, most of the rest is stored in muscle protein. Its value lies in its ability to combine with oxygen to release energy where it is needed in the body. Iron deficiency results in anaemia when the level of haemoglobin in the blood drops below 70 per cent of what it should be. The groups that need it most are menstruating women, pregnant women (the foetus needs to build up a store) and growing children. Recommended daily intakes are 6–10 mg for adult men and children up to nine years, 12–15 mg for menstruating girls and women and 15 mg for pregnant women, who are usually given an iron supplement. The best sources are liver, meat and eggs. More is absorbed if there is plenty of Vitamin C in the diet.

Na

SODIUM
Common salt, or sodium chloride, is a vital constituent for the body fluids. Too little salt, which can occasionally happen in abnormally hot weather, can result in cramps, while too much is associated with high blood pressure.

The average adult has about 200 g of salt in his body and needs about 1 g daily in food. As Western diets generally have about 5–12 g a day (much of it added to food for taste) salt deficiency is not normally a problem. Too much salt can put a strain on the kidneys which have to work to discard the excess in urine, so it is better to give young children food without salt, bland though this may seem to adult taste.

Common foods rich in salt include cheese, bacon, butter. Fresh fruits, nuts, rice and pasta contain little or no salt.

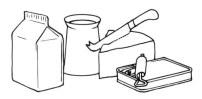

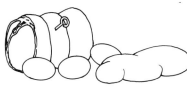

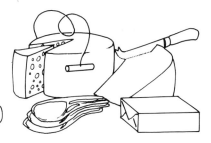

iodine (deficiency causes goitre).

One difficulty with recommending specific daily intakes of minerals is that the body absorbs minerals at different rates depending on their food source. For example, you absorb more iron from animal foods like meat than from plant-derived foods. And if it is eaten with a good source of Vitamin C then its absorption is improved. However, there is clear evidence that when food is refined, processed and cooked it loses a proportion of the minerals it held in its raw state.

Polished (white) rice, for example, has only 17 per cent of the magnesium it originally had; 25 per cent of the chromium; 25 per cent of the zinc; 73 per cent of the manganese; 62 per cent of the cobalt; and 75 per cent of the copper.

This being so, you have the best chance of obtaining enough of the minerals you need if you put an emphasis on whole and natural foods in your diet and make sure that it is as varied as possible.

P Mg K   F I Mn Zn Co Cu Cr...?

PHOSPHORUS
Like calcium, this is primarily a 'bone and teeth' mineral and that's where 85 per cent of phosphorus in the body is found. It is essential for the basic formation of the cells and for the production of energy within them. Because it is present in all living matter – both plant and animal – deficiency is virtually unknown.

MAGNESIUM
This is one of the elements in bones and needed for their development. As it is an essential ingredient in chlorophyll, the green pigment in plants, it is best found in plant-derived foods, although most foods contain it. Deficiency is rare.

POTASSIUM
An important ingredient in the fluids of the body cells which works in conjunction with sodium, potassium is found in vegetables, fruits, nuts, fish, meat and yeast extract. Deficiencies may occur following the use of diuretics or purgatives.

TRACE ELEMENTS
These are minerals found in minute quantities in the body and which are essential for health. Deficiencies in many of them are rare or unproven and the essential dietary intake of them is unknown or variable. Here are the main ones:

Fluorine – a constituent of bones and teeth, which appears to make teeth resistant to decay. In Britain the approximate intake is 1 mg a day. It is found in hard drinking water, seafood and in tea. Since 1963 the government has permitted local authorities to bring the content of fluoride in the water supply to 1 part per million because medical research suggests that people in areas with low fluoride levels in the water suffered more dental decay. Such mass medication is, however, unpopular and, as a result, many local authorities do not put fluoride in the water. Fluoride is available, however, in other forms – tablets, drops, toothpaste and in preparations applied by dentists. You can use toothpaste as you wish but ask your

dentist about other forms as they may not be necessary if you are in an area where the water has been fortified.

Iodine – a vital constituent of the hormones made by the thyroid gland. Deficiency results in goitre (swelling) in the neck as the thyroid gland swells in an effort to capture what little iodine is available. Seafood is the best source, but iodized salt is used sometimes as well. The need for iodine increases during pregnancy.

Manganese – important in the functioning of some enzymes. Plant-derived foods like cereals – especially whole grain varieties – pulses and nuts are the best sources.

Zinc – again, essential for many enzyme systems. Present especially in protein-rich foods.

Cobalt – a vital ingredient of Vitamin B12.

Copper – needed for several of the enzymes.

Chromium – needed for the utilisation of glucose.

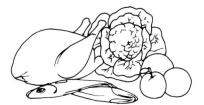

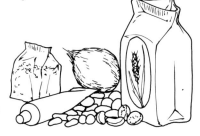

YOUR ENERGY NEEDS

Your body uses food as fuel in the same kind of way as a car uses petrol. The difference is that you put on weight if you overeat, whereas a petrol tank merely overflows if you put too much in.

So you need to know how much to eat to create the energy needed for body maintenance and physical activity without putting on (or losing) too much weight.

There is no ideal measure for this as some people have faster metabolisms than others which means they can eat more without gaining weight. Even the energy needs of an individual vary with age and activity – swimming, for example, needs ten times as much energy as sitting still. The energy value of

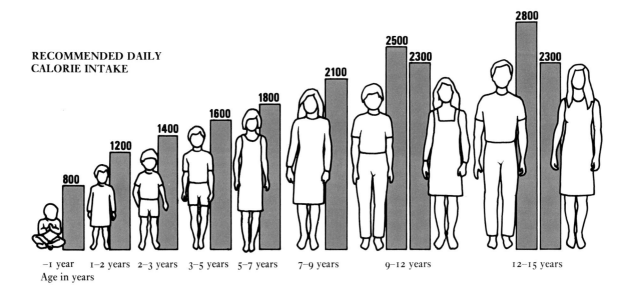

RECOMMENDED DAILY CALORIE INTAKE

800 – −1 year
1200 – 1–2 years
1400 – 2–3 years
1600 – 3–5 years
1800 – 5–7 years
2100 – 7–9 years
2500, 2300 – 9–12 years
2800, 2300 – 12–15 years

Age in years

HOW ENERGY NEEDS VARY THROUGH A SINGLE DAY
based on male office worker

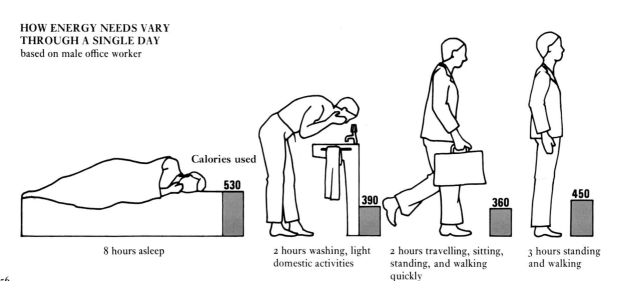

Calories used

530 — 8 hours asleep

390 — 2 hours washing, light domestic activities

360 — 2 hours travelling, sitting, standing, and walking quickly

450 — 3 hours standing and walking

food is measured in calories, each calorie being the amount of heat required to raise the temperature of 1 gramme of water by 1 degree centigrade. (As a unit of energy measurement the joule is now replacing the calorie. There are approximately 4.2 joules to a calorie.)

The calorific values of all foods are known and published and these tell you the energy value of your diet – and warn you when you are eating too much. Remember however that calories only measure energy, and are not an indication of any other nutritive value food may have.

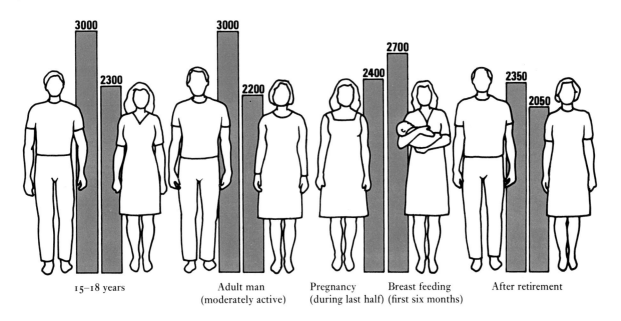

| 15–18 years | Adult man (moderately active) | Pregnancy (during last half) | Breast feeding (first six months) | After retirement |

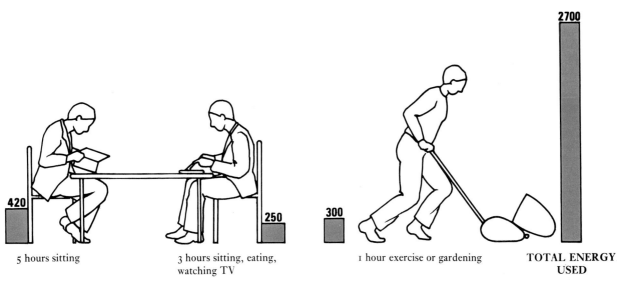

5 hours sitting   3 hours sitting, eating, watching TV   1 hour exercise or gardening   **TOTAL ENERGY USED**

EAT LESS OF THESE

The average Western diet is not perfect – typically it has too much of the wrong foods. Here we look at four categories of food that most people could cut back on to improve their health.

Here is the sugar content of some popular foods expressed in teaspoonfuls. Such figures are rough because products vary, but they serve as a warning to anyone, especially slimmers, who says 'Just one more won't hurt'.

	No. teaspoons
Ice cream ($\frac{1}{2}$ cup)	5
Sweet soda drink (6 oz)	4
Ginger ale (6 oz)	3
Average chocolate bar	7
Hot chocolate (5 oz)	6
Jam/marmalade (1 level tablespoon)	3
Canned peaches/pears (2 halves plus 1 tablespoon syrup)	3

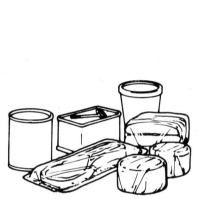

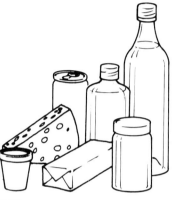

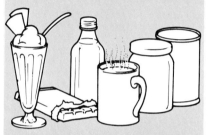

FOODS WITH ADDITIVES

A whole range of additives are put into manufactured and prepacked food to make them last longer and look nicer. For example, nitrates are used in cured and processed meat to check the growth of bacteria and give the meat an attractive pinkish colour. The use of such additives, along with prepacking and processing, makes sense in a city-based society where demands for hygiene and convenience are high. However, as there is medical evidence to suggest that excessive consumption of additives may be harmful we suggest it is sensible to use fresh, natural food wherever possible and avoid food with additives. Remember to read food labels, which, since 1970 in Britain, have had to show the ingredients of most prepacked foods in descending order of weight.

FATS

Saturated fats are mainly found in animal fats and in hardened fats. These include butter, milk, cheese, cream and some margarines. Hydrogenated fats have been hardened with hydrogen and include solid cooking fat made from vegetable oil and peanut butter (some are NOT hydrogenated). The hydrogenation process creates a fat which is saturated and more likely to increase levels of cholesterol in the blood.

ALCOHOL

Because it is absorbed quickly into the body system and goes into the water in all the cells its effects are rapid and obvious. In moderation alcohol can do no harm, but it contains virtually no nutrients and the energy it provides is in the form of empty calories.
It depresses appetite, irritates the stomach, affects the way other nutrients are used by the body and causes fat to build up in the liver.

SUGAR

It is easy to eat far more sugar than you realise because it is a hidden ingredient in so many prepacked and processed foods. Ice cream, instant puddings and biscuits are just some popular foods that usually have sugar added by manufacturers, quite apart from the obvious sugar content of confectionery, cakes, soft drinks and jams.
One result of this is that the average person in Britain eats almost 2 pounds of sugar each week.
Medical research indicates that excessive sugar is harmful to teeth and an important factor in obesity, and obese people are more likely to suffer from conditions like diabetes, gall stones and heart diseases.
Because it has little or no vitamins, minerals, fats or proteins the calories it gives you are 'empty'. Yet sugar demands a whole range of vitamins and minerals if it is to be properly absorbed by the body, including thiamin, riboflavin, pantothenic acid, phosphorus and magnesium. So it gives you little, but takes a lot.

INTRODUCTION

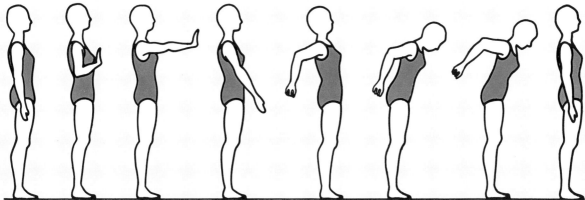

All of us need to relax – and the high incidence of stress-related diseases like atherosclerosis, raised blood pressure, and numerous psychosomatic problems seems to prove it. The trouble is that few people know how to relax and have quickly discovered that the very last way to do it is to **tell** themselves to. In the pages that follow we show how to relax successfully by becoming newly aware of the impact that stress has on our bodies by creating muscle tension, and how this can be changed. At the same time relaxation routines will help change the physical habits like shallow breathing and a hunched posture that are often the symptoms of stress. These routines are not instant cures – it is unrealistic to expect instant solutions for problems that often go back years or even decades. But follow these for two or three weeks and you will begin to notice their positive effects. Quite simply, you will enjoy life more, seem to have more energy to do the things that give you pleasure, and perhaps even be a nicer person to be with.

But remember not to strain at doing relaxation routines as you possibly strain at other things in daily living. Take them slowly, find a quiet warm room where you can practise them, and enjoy yourself.

59

HOW RELAXED ARE YOU?

HOW RELAXED ARE YOU?
The quiz that follows, like the other quizzes in this book, is non-competitive. It is based on the kind of questions, worries, complaints and symptoms that nervous, stressed people often go to doctors and healers with. If you are in doubt about any of the answers mark them 'Yes'.

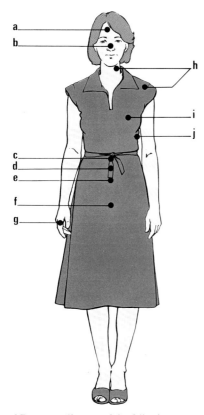

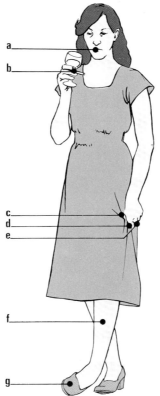

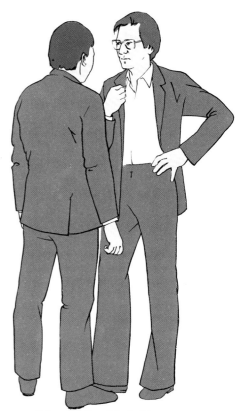

1 Do you suffer any of the following:
a migraine
b asthma
c indigestion
d flatulence
e severe menstrual pain
f constipation
g skin complaints
2 Do you sometimes have
h shoulder/neck aches
i chest pains
j back pains

3 Do you smoke or drink to 'calm your nerves'?
4 Do you do any of the following (ask someone who knows you to help with question)
a clench or grind your teeth
b chainsmoke
c tug at your clothes
d bite your nails
e twist fingers
f cross/uncross legs
g tap your feet

5 Are you dissatisfied with
a your relationships
b your job
c your life
6 If you work
a is your relationship with your superiors poor?
b do you often feel you could do a better job than your boss?
7 Is money a problem?

Count the questions with more than one answer like Nos 1 and 12 as 'Yes' if you put one 'yes' or more in them. Remember, this quiz is not a guide to specific complaints, but if you put down more than seven 'Yeses' then you are probably an unrelaxed person living with a good deal of mental and physical tension. Which means you are like the majority of people. The difference between you and them is that you have identified the problem and can do plenty about it.

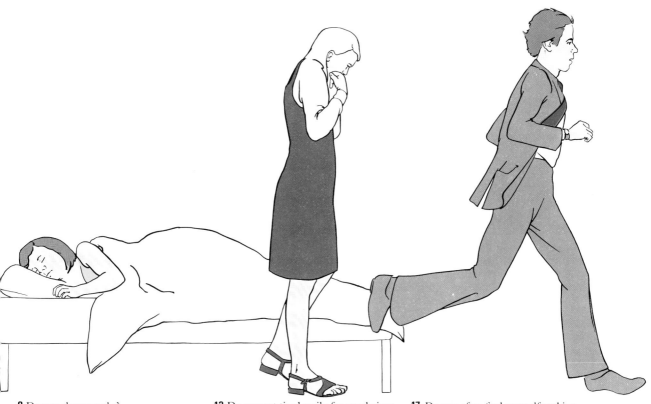

8 Do you sleep poorly?
9 Do you often wake up feeling tired and dispirited?
10 Do you take tranquillisers or sleeping pills?
11 Do you sweat at night for no obvious reason?

12 Do you get tired easily for no obvious reason?
13 Look back at the last seven days: Were you bored, miserable, wishing things would improve, or frustrated for more than four of them?
14 Are you lonely?
15 Is it true that you've done nothing – cook a meal, write a report, put up some shelves, made love – with **real joy** in the last four weeks?
16 Do others think of you as very controlled and unemotional?

17 Do you often find yourself rushing to be on time for:
a trains/buses
b work
c shops/banks
d appointments
18 Do noises make you jump?

BREATHING FOR HEALTH

Relaxed people breathe deeply, rhythmically, slowly; unrelaxed people don't. It's easy to put this to the test. Next time you get angry, or are conscious of being tense and stressed, take a look at the way you are breathing. Your breath will be shallow and fast; if you're angry it may even be so fast that you can barely control your voice. This reflects the tendency of unrelaxed people to tense their muscles – the muscles in the chest often tightening to give the familiar tension chest pain. The deep rhythmic breathing of the truly relaxed person is not merely a sign of being relaxed; it is also a **cause** of health and well being in itself. The trouble with suddenly starting breathing exercises and taking lots of deep breaths is that it turns a process that should be utterly natural and unconscious into a conscious effort. Indeed, relaxed healthy people are rarely conscious of the fact that they are deep breathers. For this reason the routines that follow are not daily exercises to do for ever more. They are designed principally to make you conscious, perhaps for the first time, of how important deep breathing is, and how good it can feel. They will also make you aware of how shallow much of your breathing often is. If you do them you will find that relaxation comes automatically after a surprisingly short while, and that quite soon deep relaxed breathing will become routine to you. At that point you will have no need of conscious deliberate exercises showing you how to breathe and only use them occasionally as a trigger for deep relaxation. As with all the routines and exercises in this book, do them somewhere quiet and peaceful, where you can concentrate solely on them. Do not try to do these routines all at once – take it slowly and enjoy them.

DEEP NATURAL BREATHING

This is one of the simplest, most enjoyable relaxation routines you can do. If you are angry, tense, overtired, or just depressed try it out and see how much better you feel afterwards.

– Lie on the floor (only on a bed if it is really firm) and stretch out slowly. Your feet should be slightly apart, with toes and ankles limp, the arms clear of the body with the palms facing the ceiling. Picture for a moment something that is pleasant and calming – perhaps the sea, or trees in sunlight in a gentle wind. Become slowly conscious of your breathing, watching it as if it were someone else's breathing.

– Now feel each breath enter the nose, travel to the back of the throat and down into the lungs. As it enters your lungs feel your diaphragm rising but NOT YOUR CHEST. Put your hands for a moment on your diaphragm, feeling it rise with each breath. Let each breath become deeper and slower.

– Do this ten times, letting the breaths come naturally. As you exhale feel the breath leave the body, and your trunk almost sinking into the floor. There should be a moment of empty stillness before slowly, rhythmically, the new breath starts again and your abdomen (REPEAT: NOT YOUR CHEST) starts to rise again.

– Let each breath come at its own pace. DO NOT try to control the rate of breathing – being conscious only of its depth.

– Now forget your breathing for a moment and visualise different parts of your body – your feet, your legs, your buttocks, the small of your back, your shoulders, neck and face. Feel them warm and relaxed.

– As you come to each part feel it through one breath cycle, seeing how each part of your body responds to each breath. This will be more noticeable with parts of your body near your lungs – your back, shoulders, neck and the small of your back. But after a time you will begin to feel the 'breath movement' in every part of your body.

Now return to your breathing and passively watch four more breath cycles. Finally, stretch and, if you feel like it, yawn or sigh. Get up very slowly and indulgently as if you have all the time in the world. Sit up or kneel for three or four breaths before standing up.

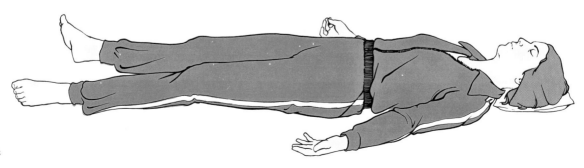

WHAT DEEP BREATHING DOES
1 It fully clears the lungs of the waste products picked up from de-oxygenated blood as it passes through them.
2 It involves continual full use of a whole range of muscles in the chest, diaphragm and back. If, like millions of people, you have long been a shallow breather, then these muscles will have weakened just as other muscles in the arms and legs grow weak if you don't use them.
3 Full, deep breathing has a massaging effect on organs like the stomach, kidneys, intestines, sex organs and bladder.
4 Proper breathing is through the nose, which means that air is cleaned and warmed before it reaches the lungs. Tense, shallow breathers often breathe through their mouths.

ALTERNATE BREATHING
This routine takes less than a minute but is very relaxing – and clears the head. It's good to do when you are feeling muggy. Sit back on your haunches with your spine erect. (Or you can do this sitting in a chair.) Rest your left hand on your thigh. Place the index and forefinger of your right hand on the top of your nose between your eyes. Your thumb should now be on the right nostril, your ring finger by the left. Now close the right nostril by pressing your thumb against it. Breathe in through your left nostril slowly and deeply. Now press your ring finger against the left nostril, closing it. Release the right nostril and breathe out through it. Breathe in again through your right nostril, reversing the process and then out through your left . . . and so on. Do this eight times. It is important to keep your back straight and head well up – not bent deep into your chest.

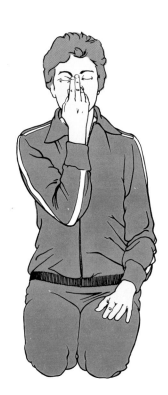

ACTION BREATHING
This is a way of turning something like drying yourself after a bath, dressing in the morning, even hanging out the washing, into an exercise in breathing relaxation. All you do is to perform the task much slower than normal, breathing deeply and rhythmically as you do it. Let the rhythm of each breath dictate the pace at which you perform the task. Stop for a moment sometimes just to enjoy the refreshing depth of your breathing. One advantage of this kind of routine is that it 'informalises' good breathing, making it the natural part of living it should really be. Other relaxation exercises that follow will show you how to feel the breath of life with your whole body.

THE SEVEN BREATHS
Done slowly and concentratedly this exercise is very relaxing. Never try to do it twice running. The best time is at night, **immediately** before bed. In other words make sure you've locked up, put the milk bottles out, set the central heating, got rid of the cat or anything else that will disturb the deep rhythm the routine creates.
– Lie on your back on the floor as in the first routine.
– Let your breathing slowly develop into a nice deep unforced rhythm. This should take one or two minutes.
– Now think of each breath as, literally, a breath of life, drawing cleanliness, light, energy, health into you.
– You are going to take seven breaths, with each one concentrating on one part of the body. Imagine that each breath comes through that part of the body – some people like to do this as if the breath is light entering the body, but you may prefer to visualise it as the flow of water, or simply as a current of cool clean air. Each inhalation is through the nose, each exhalation through the mouth.
– Now breathe in through the back of the head slowly and deeply. Feel the energy flow from the back of your head down to your abdomen. Hold the breath for the count of five and then release it (DON'T force it, let it take its own pace) through the mouth. Feel the stillness at the end of the breath for a second or two.
– Now breathe in through the forehead and follow the same routine.
– Now the base of the brain.
– Now the abdomen.
– Now the sexual organs.
– Now the soles of the feet. These are the seven breaths.
Now take an eighth breath in through the whole body. As you breathe it out feel the total relaxation in the body. Get up slowly and go to bed.

RELAXATION ROUTINE 1

These two pages are an invitation to experiment with sensuality, to become more aware of the feelings and physical sensations in your body. If you have spent some days doing our breathing routines it is an experiment you have already started, perhaps without realising it. When you are breathing in a deep rhythmic way, for example, you may become aware of enjoying the movement of the muscles in the abdomen, chest and back. If you are not quite sure about this feeling try it now by doing the first breathing routine. Feel the way the abdomen rises and falls, sense the pleasurable feel of your expanding lungs, and the release and calm you feel as you breathe out. Almost certainly too you will have had a sense of warmth doing these routines – 'a golden glow' as some describe it when they first feel it. Such feelings are an important step towards learning the habits of deep relaxation. Just as for a time you need to become unnaturally aware of your breathing, so it helps to become conscious of how your arms and legs, hands and feet, chest and back feel when they are tensed or relaxed. It may be strange to discover that after decades of living in your body you probably rarely respond

GRAND TOUR OF THE BODY

Try this experiment. Lie down some-where warm and firm – a carpeted floor is ideal. Lie with arms clear of the body, palms facing upwards, legs a little apart with the feet loose and falling away from the body, head supported by no more than one pillow, eyes closed. Breathe slowly and deeply for a minute or so. Now start a mental exploration of the way your body feels – really a sensual Grand Tour of your own body. Remember all the time – YOU ARE IN NO HURRY. How do your feet (**1**) feel? Are they cold, warm or hot? Are your toes (**2**) relaxed or tense? Do they ache very slightly? Wiggle your feet and ankles about a bit if necessary to get a better sense of how they feel. Spend no more than a minute on each part. Now move your ankles (**3**). Can you feel one better than the other (people can often feel the right side of their body better than the left)? Move on to your calves (**4**). If you're a little tired they may well have a light ache about them. Then your knees (**5**). So to your thighs (**6**) and

buttocks (**7**), asking yourself all the time what sensations you feel – heavy, light, tired, glowing, cold . . . and so on. Note areas which seem to send you no signals as if you cannot feel them.
Now – start with the small of your back (**8**), trying to move up to your shoulders (**9**) by really sensing the feel of the spine. This is often quite difficult because many people have acquired stiff, insensitive backs. Now your arms (**10**) and hands (**11**) – which part is harder to feel, which easiest? You may be surprised at how much sense of strain or discomfort there is in your hands. Switch to your stomach (**12**), abdomen (**13**) and chest (**14**), feeling the muscle movement involved with each breath, enjoying the sense of warmth and calm that follows each exhalation.
Travel finally to your neck (**15**), gently moving it from side to side as you do so, to become aware of it. Then to your mouth (**16**) – are your teeth and tongue tense? And finally your face – how do your eyes feel (**17**), your cheeks (**18**), your forehead (**19**)? Enjoy this Grand Tour

of your body for fifteen minutes or so, noting which areas you find it easiest to feel, which ones feel uncomfortable, and which ones you get little response from at all. Finally, see if you can get a sense of awareness of your whole body – feel its weight bearing you down – your hands, feet and shoulders in particular may almost seem to want to sink into the floor. Feel its warmth and finish the journey with another minute or two of deep rhythmic breathing. It's a good idea to make a note immediately afterwards of what you felt: which parts of your body you felt most easily; which were uncomfortable; which were warm; which seemed insensitive and unresponsive: write it down and put it somewhere safe. Even better, do the exercise with someone else – talking your way through your body and getting him or her to write down what you say. Initial embarrassment will soon go – but insist that your helper stays quiet and silent through the process, not intruding his or her thoughts on yours.

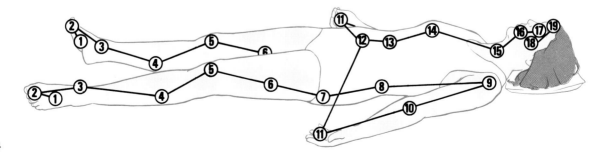

fully to the range of sensory messages it sends to you. If you are tense you cut yourself off from them. One of the effects of stress is to rob you of enjoying the feeling of health in whole areas of the body by putting them under continual and desensitising tension.

We all sense that our physical stamina and emotional state fluctuate so that we have good times and bad, times when we say 'Everything's gone wrong today and I really feel under the weather', or 'I've been so full of energy today it has been incredible'. Women recognise such rhythms, and learn to live with them far better than men because of the inescapable physical fact of their menstrual cycle. But, as we have seen, men have their emotional and physical rhythms too. The levels of sex hormones in the urine of men, for example, appear to fluctuate on a monthly basis; and industrial psychologists have charted the emotional ups and downs of male workers and found they fall into a cyclical pattern.

HOW STRESS TENSES UP YOUR MUSCLES

Head Moves forward – jutting out stiffly if you are afraid or angry, hanging down into the chest if you are in pain or sad. Neck muscles rigid and stiff.

Face Teeth clench together as jaw clamps tight. Lips are tense, the tongue tense and rigid and raised to the roof of the mouth. Brows are furrowed and eyes screwed up and strained or open wide.

Breathing The chest muscles are tense, the breathing quick and shallow. The outward breath especially is quick and incomplete, failing to empty the lungs fully. You may breathe through your mouth. Tense muscles like this quickly tire and for this reason an unrelaxed person often complains of aches and pains, especially in the back, shoulders and neck.

Arms Upper arms tighten into the chest as you lift your shoulders towards your ears and hold them there. Elbows stiff and locked.

Hands Thumb and fingers curl tensely, clenching each other or even forming a fist. Arms tighten into your chest. You grasp anything you are holding (telephone, car steering wheel) tightly, or twist and intertwine fingers.

Trunk Tense and rigid and often hunched stiffly forward at the hips, straining at the small of the back and shoulders.

Legs If you are sitting down your legs are crossed (often again and again), the top foot tense and pointing upwards. You may sit on the edge of your chair. If you are standing you may still cross your legs over each other or move about a lot.

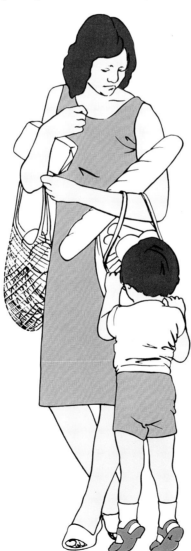

HOW TO DEAL WITH TENSION

An unrelaxed person is unlikely to display all these reactions at once, but you can usually see two or three of them. Now try this experiment: Run through the list above, deliberately putting your muscles into the tense positions described: cross your legs, clench your hands, stiffen your neck and so on. Hold the position for a moment or two. How do you feel? **Now do the exact opposite.**

Deliberately stretch your hands, loosen your neck by rolling it, stretch your trunk, deepen your breathing and so on. If you are sitting down and feel it would be better to lie down and really stretch out, do so. When you've done all the opposites, go limp. Now ask yourself how you feel . . .

If you feel much more relaxed, as you almost certainly do, you have demonstrated an important fact to yourself. You **can** alter your feelings of tension and relaxation by consciously changing your muscles' positions. In the following pages we show how to do this properly for the different parts of the body. But by opening up your feelings about your body's tensions you have already taken the first step.

RELAXATION ROUTINE 2

The relaxation routines that follow are designed for specific parts of the body – the arms, the legs and the trunk. Many of them you can do anywhere, using a few moments of a busy day to give your body a break. But to start with it is a good idea to practise them somewhere quiet and calm. Some can only be done lying down – the best position for relaxation routines. Do the others lying down as well where that applies, but also practise them sitting and standing because that is often the only way you can do them in normal unrelaxed daily life.

You will find that the effects of these routines go deeper the more you do them. Regard these routines as habit creators, not instant cures for every ache and pain. Many of our physical tensions are the result of habits created over years of misusing our bodies – it takes a long time to change these habits. But it is a consolation to know that the body's ability to heal itself is very great, so that once you start treating it right it responds quickly – although rarely overnight.

ELBOWS If you are sitting, place your palms on the table in front, or on the arms of a chair (or your thighs will do) and swing your elbows up and away from the body, keeping your hands on the table or chair. The movement will only be a matter of inches but you will feel a pull in the elbows. If you are lying on the floor put your hands on your hips, rest your elbows on the floor and push them away from the body but keep them on the floor. Again, the real movement will be slight.

THIGHS Start by sitting in a chair. Massage with your fingertips all around the area above the knee, feeling the sensations of release travelling up your thighs. Now, resting your legs and thighs on the balls of your feet, let them go loose and shake them as if they were jelly.

FEET Arch your feet away from your body. If you are lying down this is straightforward; but if sitting in a chair it means raising your legs onto the **underside** of your toes which will splay out. If you go onto the tips of your toes the effect is not so powerful.

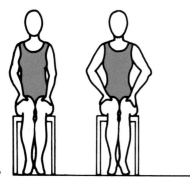

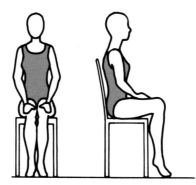

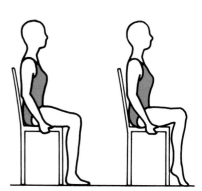

HANDS – Massage both sides of the tissue between where the thumb joins the hand (**1**). Do this firmly but gently for a minute each side.
– Massage each joint of each finger, again quite firmly. Pull each finger back so that you feel a gentle stretching tension down its length and hold for a moment (**2**).
Place your palm flat against a wall at shoulder height so that the arms are stretched straight out. Feel the tension along the length of the hand and arm. Let your arms fall to your sides limply; shake the hand as if it is a rag at the end of your arm. Do this with both hands.
– Finally, stretch both hands in front of you, arching them out of the clenched curled position they often adopt (**3**).

TOES Like the fingers, they're often forgotten. Get into the habit of massaging each individual joint after a bath – sitting on the floor is the best position. Also massage the areas 'a' and 'b' as shown in diagram below. **Whenever possible** take your shoes off. None of these routines should be forced – indeed you should never **force** your muscles or your body to do anything. But nor should they be done so gently that you feel no pulling.

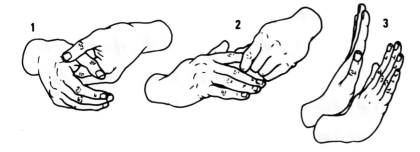
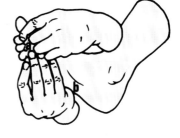

SHOULDERS If lying on the ground pull the shoulders down towards the feet away from the ears. Do not hunch them forward or pull them back. Hold them for a brief moment in the new position and then relax.

Rest your fingertips on your shoulders and breathe deeply into your abdomen slowly two or three times. Then, on an inhalation, arc your elbows out and up from the body until you can feel the pull of muscles through your back and chest, keeping your fingers on your shoulder. As you exhale, relax the arms and let them fall loosely at your sides. Breathe deeply a couple more times, feeling the release in your shoulder muscles.

LEGS Lying on the ground, stretch your legs out in front for a moment, and go limp. Now, bending the foot at the ankle towards the knee and keeping the legs straight, raise one leg gently about 6 inches off the ground. You will feel a pull up your calf. Lower your leg to the floor and repeat with the other. Do this twice for each leg.

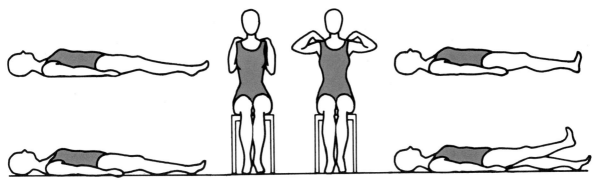

RELAXATION ROUTINE 3

These routines will help you relax key parts of the body that become tense when you are strained, and whose tension may have become a habit. The one area not covered is the lower back. This is covered by the next two relaxer exercises, and by the routines described later.

YOUR HEAD Few people really believe that the head is quite heavy – about 11 pounds in fact. No wonder your head, neck and shoulders so often ache under tension. – Lie on the floor, or lean back comfortably in a seat with support for your head, and press your head into the floor or chair. Hold for a moment. Relax and let the floor or chair take the weight. This simple routine is a surprisingly effective way of relaxing the muscles that support the head.

YOUR BODY This is best done lying down. Press your body into the floor – calves, thighs, buttocks, back, shoulders, head, arms. Hold the position for a moment only and then relax and **as you do** so feel the real weight of your body sinking into the floor. In short, let the floor take the whole weight. This is sometimes difficult at first as we are used to tensing muscles as if ready for action. But do this over a few days and you will find yourself releasing more and more of your own weight for the floor or chair to support.

The last two routines are exercises which combine several of these techniques, creating an effective way of relaxing your whole body. They are best done in the early evening when your body is likely to be more supple than at other times of the day but not too tired. Try to do them at least two hours after eating. This means that if you work all day a good time is just before your evening meal; use it as a way of helping to rid your body of the physical tensions it has picked up through the day.

RELAXER ONE

1 Stand with your spine straight, arms hanging loosely at sides, and feet together.
2 Raise your hands slowly, touching your chest just above each breast, palms facing outwards.
3 Straighten your arms gently in front of you, keeping hands at right angles to your arms. You should feel a pull running through your hands, forearms, elbows and upper arms.
4 Swing the arms slowly behind you and lower them until you can interlock the fingers.
5 Lean **gently** backwards a few inches, keeping your arms high but without

straining. Breathe twice in and out deeply and slowly. Keep the legs straight. Do this slowly, never straining.
6 With fingers still interlocked behind you, lean gently forward, relaxing the neck muscles so that the head hangs forward.
7 Bring arms above back and hold them as high as is comfortable. Do this slowly, never straining. Keep your legs straight. Breathe in and out slowly four times.
8 Very gently return to a vertical position, letting your hands swing back loosely to your side. Do this routine three times in succession but rest each time, and do not start again until you feel ready to.

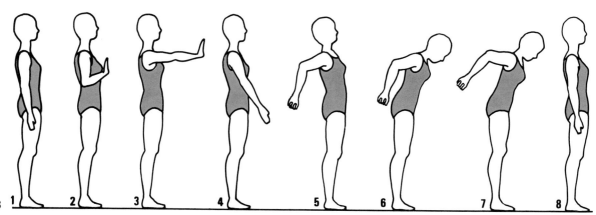

YOUR FACE People rarely notice that when they are stressed they clench their jaws and force the tongue to the roof of the mouth. This easily becomes a habit. So now do the opposite . . . Open your mouth and pull your lower jaw down, as if yawning. (**1**) Do this slowly and hold it for a moment. Now relax, letting your lower teeth hang clear of your upper teeth but bringing your lips together. (**2**) The jaw should be slack so that if you shake your head you can feel it loose in your mouth. Press your tongue to the floor of your mouth and hold for a moment. (**3**) Relax. Let your tongue hang loose so that it stays in the middle of your mouth (**4**).

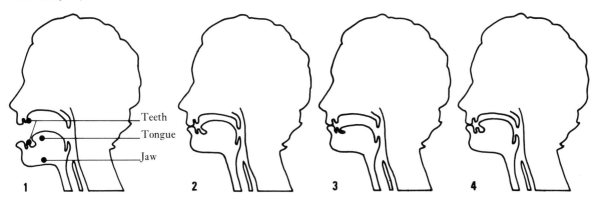

RELAXER TWO

1 Sit on the floor with your legs straight and your hands resting loosely on your thighs.
2 Raise your arms slowly in an arc until your fingertips touch above your head with your arms bent very slightly at each elbow. Turn the palms of your hands towards your toes.
3 Bend backwards very gently two or three inches and hold the position for three slow breaths.

4 Very slowly bend forward, bringing your hands down to rest on your legs just below the knees. Keep your legs straight but relaxed.
5 Bend head and trunk slowly forward WITHOUT STRAIN. It does not matter if you can bend forward only very slightly; people have very different capacities for this movement and how far you go (or don't go) will not affect the exercise's total relaxation effect. Hold this position for four breaths and sit up vertically again, hands placed gently again on thighs.
6 Finally, lie back on the floor and, with a head support if you prefer it, breathe deeply into your diaphragm five times or so. Get up slowly.
REMEMBER WITH BOTH THESE RELAXER EXERCISES THAT YOU MUST MAKE ALL MOVEMENTS VERY SLOWLY AND BE GENTLE WITH YOURSELF. NEVER, NEVER STRAIN.

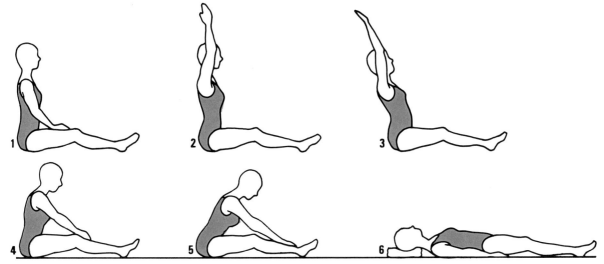

MEDITATE FOR HEALTH

The best way to approach meditation is to do it. Try not to think about ideas you have of its mystery, its difficulty, its rites and secrets. Simply do it. Why? Perhaps because of curiosity about its popularity, or interest in the research that has been carried out into its effects on the mind and body. The latter suggests that after quite a short period, weeks of doing it rather than years, your breathing slows down, your heart rate falls, blood pressure falls, your metabolism slows and there is decreased 'nervous activity'. You don't have to believe any of this, though such research has been done by a wide spread of reputable doctors and scientists in several countries, to benefit. But don't expect to see visions, flashing lights or golden waterfalls. Indeed don't expect anything out of the ordinary at all – except a slow building-up of a calmer, more objective view of things and yourself.

WHERE TO BEGIN

Some practical suggestions may help: Choose a quiet room where you know you will not be disturbed. Lighting should be subdued – a candle is ideal, placed behind you where its flickering will not distract you.
How do you know when your time's up?

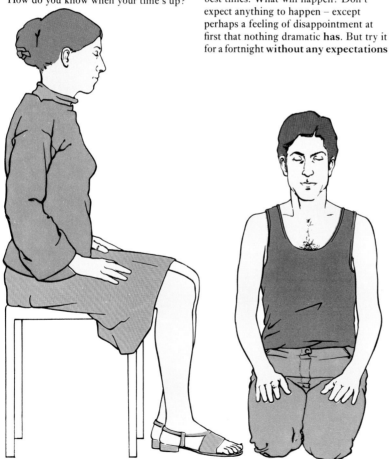

At the beginning it may help to have a clock, the quieter the better, placed where you can see it without moving. After a while you won't need it. Do not meditate within two hours of eating, preferably longer. First thing in the morning, or last thing at night are the best times. What will happen? Don't expect anything to happen – except perhaps a feeling of disappointment at first that nothing dramatic **has**. But try it for a fortnight **without any expectations** and then see how you feel about it. Like many people you may soon find you look forward to your short period of meditation without quite knowing why. Perhaps it's because this is the first time for a long while, perhaps ever, that you have sat quietly, shedding the jumble of thoughts that normally crowd the mind, carried along on one emotional, nervous current after another. Perhaps it is because it is so peaceful giving yourself the freedom not to have to respond to those thoughts by concentrating on something as simple (and all-important) as breathing. You will find your own answers.

HOW TO BEGIN

1 Sit in a chair or kneel on the floor **comfortably** – do not try to adopt a difficult cross-legged position if it is uncomfortable, though it may prove the best position eventually.
2 Close your eyes and slow down! Use some of the breathing techniques already described; the process should not take more than one or two minutes. Don't try to force the relaxation – it will come automatically.
3 Now, breathing through your nose, count each exhalation. One . . . two . . . three . . . four. Then go back to the beginning again. Don't hurry it, or force it. Simply let each breath count itself.
4 Do this for fifteen minutes. As you do it think only about your breathing. Other thoughts will come into your mind but be passive towards them, not getting involved in them, letting them evaporate. Simply keep on counting your breaths . . . one, two, three, four.
5 When you have finished, stay where you are quietly. Open your eyes slowly. Get up gently. Repeat this once a day, or twice if you can find time.

There is no one right way to meditate. Adepts themselves vary the method they use, and so should you. Relaxation is a by-product of meditation, never its aim. In its pursuit you may well find that many of the things that cause you stress or tension no longer seem so important. If you want to pursue it there are now many books and teachers to choose from.

CHOOSE YOUR OWN WAY

There are many other methods of meditation, each reflecting the nature of the culture and philosophy from which they come. To know more about them you will need to take instruction, study and perhaps go on a course. But here are some of the techniques you may come across, which you can try for yourself. Remember there is no one 'right' way to meditate, so experiment!

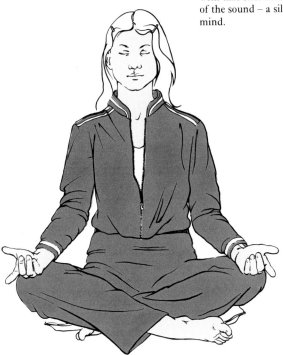

Use sound If you've ever listened to Gregorian chant, or plainsong, and perhaps hummed with it, you'll know how sound can calm you and fill you with peace. Such chanting is in fact a form of meditation and prayer. Some people find it helpful to meditate using a sound such as aummmmmm or ommmmmm or even two or three vowel sounds together: ooooooooooh aaaaaaaaaaaaaaaah, eeeeeeeeeee. At first it feels strange and you may be self-conscious, but persevere for two or three minutes each day. You will probably find that one sound suits you best – so stick with that one. Also you can simply think of the sound – a silent sound in your mind.

Use pictures Find a picture or illustration that gives you pleasant relaxed thoughts. Sitting comfortably, let your thoughts wander into it, concentrating on it alone. If other thoughts intrude return your attention to the picture and let them slip away.

Use a mantra A mantra is a letter, word, sound or phrase repeated continually in meditation to the exclusion of thoughts. It may be specially chosen for you if, for example, you follow a specific school such as Transcendental Meditation. Repeating a word with good associations such as 'love', 'tree', 'peace', or 'God' silently or aloud is a meditation. Associated words or ideas will come into your mind – that's fine, but after a few seconds return to the mantra.

Use a prayer Repetition and concentration are characteristics of many meditations, and prayers are often used for this purpose. The Christian 'Jesus Prayer' is just such a prayer, repeated again and again. Its English form is simply 'Lord Jesus Christ, Son of God, have mercy on me a sinner'.

The Lord's Prayer is another, indeed it is really a series of mantras. You don't have to be any denomination, or even a Christian, to feel a greater peace for repeating it slowly, concentrating on each phrase in it, twice a day.

PLAN FOR RELAXATION

We let habits run our lives; but too often they are bad habits. We eat poor food, we get too little exercise, we 'relax' into tense postures. The difficulty is that once habits are established they may be hard to break. Every home and office has what we call tension points – small areas of bad planning or inefficiency which may cause you, and your family or office colleagues, unnecessary tension. Have you got a do-it-yourself job somewhere in the house that has never quite been

YOUR HOME

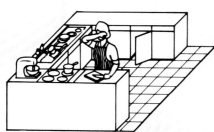 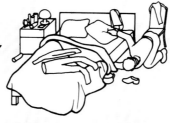 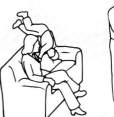 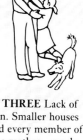

TENSION POINT ONE The way you work may reflect tensions you feel and cause you more. Do you grip kitchen utensils very tightly when you work with them? Do you give yourself backache by the force you put into sweeping or washing things down? Do you hurry jobs so much that you do them poorly and get little pleasure from them? Have another look at our relaxation routine and try doing jobs that way.

TENSION POINT TWO Untidiness is a major tension point in many homes. A home does not have to be in a mess to be untidy. If you can't find things easily, if you have no set place for dirty laundry, if your bedside table isn't big enough for the things you keep by the bed, if your wardrobe doesn't hold all your clothes properly, then you have an untidy situation. It is **worth** making time to sort it all out.

TENSION POINT THREE Lack of privacy causes tension. Smaller houses mean less privacy and every member of a family – especially the mother – needs to be alone sometimes. Privacy is not simply being alone in a room – it is also not being disturbed, a rather different thing. People need time alone without the intrusion of noise (television, record player) or personal pressures ('I'll need your help in ten minutes' time'). Ask yourself and your family what tension points they can think of in your home and remember that however unreasonable someone's complaint may seem, the fact of making it means it deserves to be taken seriously.

HELP YOURSELF WITH BETTER ROUTINES

– If there's something you want to see or listen to on radio or TV, organise your household jobs around it. Cooking in the middle of a TV serial you like watching causes tension, so plan around it. Running the dishwasher in the middle of a quiet sit-down isn't much fun either.
– Make a regular routine of clearing drawers, lumber rooms, garages and attics. Everyone accumulates junk, but there's no need to keep it for a lifetime. It is a tension creator because it makes it hard to find things.
– Surveys show that bedmaking is one of the least-liked jobs in the home. Continental quilts (duvets) really are a time saver.
– Have a break every day from your home and try to make it something more constructive (and cheaper) than going shopping. This is hard for mothers of small children – but even gardening in bad weather or coffee with a neighbour is preferable to staying in your own home day after day.
– Viewing figures show the average adult watches about 3 hours of TV **every day**. This means that they are sitting in a room, probably with poor ventilation, and in poorly designed seats, physically inactive and mentally strained. Try **not** watching for just two days running, and do something instead that you always said you were going to do but never quite got round to.

finished? That's a tension point. Has your desk never been really sorted out for months? That's another tension point. Such things are rarely serious in themselves but, like the Chinese water torture, they are cumulative. A series of small hassles through the day can create very real stress and tension. We can't identify your own tension points for you, but the ideas below suggest where you should start looking and demonstrate how easy it is to eliminate tension creators.

YOUR OFFICE

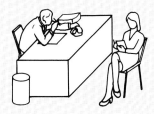

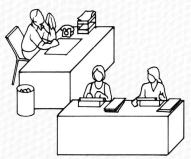

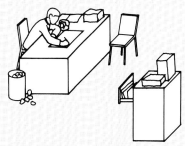

TENSION POINT ONE Your chair and desk. People put up for years on end with chairs and desks which don't suit them. Play around with the height of your chair and see if a taller or lower one would suit you better. Chairs with arms give more support, chairs with high backs support the head and neck. Desk positions can be changed to reduce tension too – don't face the light, avoid a position where there is a continual traffic of people behind you, choose a position which makes it easier to work with the people you need to talk to.

TENSION POINT TWO Room temperature and noise. Research shows that when levels of temperature and noise are too high work deteriorates because people are under stress. Optimum temperature ranges vary with different people so this may be difficult to change – but it is worth trying.

TENSION POINT THREE If you never seem to have time to think in your job then the chances are that you are not properly organised. Some jobs never end and there's not much you can do about it. But many jobs can be kept in control day by day – letters cleared, orders chased up, projects progressed: it's just a matter of routine. Be prepared to spend a weekend working out the better routines and even clearing back correspondence so that you can feel on top of the job. Coming in early for a period may pay off too.

IMPROVE YOUR WORKING DAY

Few office workers ever exploit the many ways they can relieve the tension of their jobs . . .
– The telephone. Next time you pick up a telephone watch how you handle it. You probably grip the receiver too tightly, push it against your ear, hunch over it, sit forward in your chair as you speak, begin shallow breathing. In short, you display all the classic physical signs of tension. Try sitting back, breathing deeply and holding the phone a little away from your ear. Deliberately relax your hands, arms, legs and feet (pages 66–67) as you talk.

– Find exercise points where you work, or while travelling to work. Climb stairs, walk the final tube station or bus-stop, see if there is a swimming bath or gymnasium nearby. Get some exercise every day.
– Plan your office holidays well in advance. Try not to leave too much of a gap between them – especially in the dreary period between Christmas and Easter, and in the autumn if you have a main midsummer holiday. Even if it is only a long weekend away it pays off.
– Play the stress-watch game by watching others in the office for some of the stress

signs outlined in the quiz on pages 60–61. And watch yourself as well.
– Create a personal environment in your office, or around your desk if you are in an open-plan office. Pictures, plants, personal effects help create an environment in which you can relax. Think carefully about colours too; those at the red end of the spectrum are exciting and unrelaxing, while colours near the blue end are relaxing.
– Try to get out of your office building at least once a day. The fresh air and change will do you good and help in your relaxation programme.

ORGANISE HOME AND OFFICE

We live life in units of one day at a time. A series of rushed, disorganised, harried days creates a tense, unrelaxed life. It's a fact that healthy relaxed people do not live like that although they often live **fuller, busier** lives than the average person. They have learned to do two things: to value their time, and to enjoy every minute of it. There is probably no quicker way of creating the beginnings of a healthy relaxed life than simply sitting down and looking critically at the way you run your day-to-day life. Don't try to make a new life plan, or organise the next twelve months. Just look critically at the way you spent the last seven days and see what you can learn to improve the way you propose running the next seven.

SIX SIMPLE THINGS WORTH TRYING

The following six ideas may sound too simple to be worthwhile – at first. But just try them and see.
1 Set your clock or watch five minutes fast.
2 Be early for trains and appointments for a week.
3 Clear your kitchen before you go to bed and lay breakfast ahead.
4 Clear your desk before you leave the office.
5 Tidy and clean inside your car once a week.
6 Have an in-tray for bills and household paper work where you can see it.

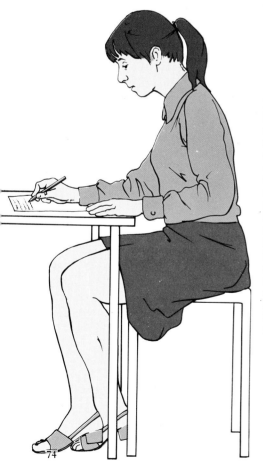

MAKE A START TODAY

Start **now** by setting time aside – you'll need a couple of hours – sometime in the next two or three days to plan the week ahead. If you're married arrange to do it with your spouse – you'll learn a lot and both be involved; if you've got children make sure they are in bed. Turn the television off, take the phone off the hook, sit down with plenty of paper at a table where you can write comfortably. Naive? Well, run through the list of ideas for a more relaxed day that follows and there's certain to be one area where you can improve things and end up more relaxed. Jot your own ideas down as they come to you and then reorganise them into a system – setting aside more time next week to review progress.

PLAN YOUR DAY
Simple advice, but too few do it. At any one moment the average person has at least ten, probably nearer twenty, things he ought to be doing shortly – like pay a couple of bills, check a train time, prepare for an interview in two days' time, buy a spare car part, file papers, answer two letters . . . and so on. These are all things that **must** be done, so why make them tension-creators by leaving them until the last moment? One method that works is to list things you must do in a pocket-sized notebook as they come up – and then cross them off as you do them. Revise the list every two days. A task written down is one less to remember. No two people plan their day the same way but there **is** one general principle: it pays to spend five minutes in the morning or evening planning the day ahead. That's the time to go through your list of things to do and work out what you need to do and when to do them. It's a discipline that takes a little practice, but it pays.

DON'T RUSH BREAKFAST This is
the most important meal of the day,
psychologically and physically. Rush it
and your mind and body are tense right
from the word go; take it slowly and you
are ready prepared for the day.

KNOW YOUR RHYTHMS On pages
18–19 we showed how biological rhythms
affect your life. Read those pages again,
remember that it pays in terms of time,
energy and relaxation to know your
personal rhythms.
If you find you do brain work better in
the morning plan to do it then; if you're
physically more 'awake' in the evening,
aim to fit in your exercise routine then,
and so on. Most women feel a little tired
or keyed-up just before or during
menstruation – plan ahead accordingly.
If your normal sleeping pattern is likely
to be disturbed for more than one night,
plan for it. It can happen when you go
on holiday, or perhaps when someone
comes visiting. Expect there to be
periods in a month when you feel
physically low and pamper yourself then.

**ARE YOU INEFFICIENT AT YOUR
WORK?** Whether our job is the house
and children or in an office, most of us
know whether we could be more
efficient. If the thought nags at us then
we probably could organise things better.
And it's often the basics that can be
improved. Thousands of commuters, for
example, never work out whether they
travel to the office in the most efficient,
healthy way. Unlikely? Well, one survey
showed that for short one- or two-stop
bus journeys it's often quicker to walk,
yet few do so. Travelling can be
significantly easier earlier or later than
normal rush hour – the new 'flexitime'
system shows that such routines can be
negotiated.

GIVE YOURSELF A DAILY BREAK
You need a break by yourself **every** day.
Most of us are surrounded by people,
whether family, workmates or neighbours.
That's fine, but twenty-four hours a day,
every day? That's unreasonable. Try to
plan a personal break for yourself each
day – a time perhaps to try some of the
breathing or meditation routines in this
section. Surprisingly, many families
object, even if only indirectly, if one of
their members pops into the spare room
to be alone for ten minutes, so you may
need to be tough about it. But the
first couple of times are the hardest.
This is especially important for mothers
of small children and something their
husbands – who have more opportunity
for a break – should be prepared to cater
for. They will benefit. The same applies
to executives working in open-plan offices
who often end up sharing lunch with
business colleagues every day as well.
Eight to ten hours a day continuously
with workmates is too much, and a break
will pay. Most towns have churches
which are quiet and open at lunchtime –
try popping in and sitting down for a
few minutes, if only once a week.

VALUE YOUR TIME Unrelaxed
people often complain that they **never
have time.**
If this is so there are two possible
reasons: either they are doing too much
or they are doing it inefficiently.
There is nothing wrong with deadlines –
indeed they are often needed to give the
impetus to get things done – but there is
something wrong if deadlines control
your life to the point where they create
tension. The solution lies first in
convincing yourself that your priorities
need to change so that the **first** priority
is that each day gives you time to do the
things you need to do at the pace at
which you can enjoy them and do them
properly. This really is important because
you can (and many do) rush yourself into
bad jobs, poor relationships, a frustrated
life, and an early grave.

PREPARE FOR THE WORST
Everyone has tricky situations to face,
particularly with people. This is almost
inevitable in any responsible job, and
surprisingly common at home as well.
Interviews, meetings with solicitors, bank
managers, returning faulty goods,
irregular once-only bills – they crop up
all the time. One technique for handling
them, very effective with personal
confrontations, is to visualise the
situation before and work out your
response to the different possibilities.
Really ask yourself 'what **will** I say or
do if . . .' Unresolved imaginings are a
major cause of tension in busy people,
and often a totally unnecessary effort.
This approach not only makes you
relaxed but usually makes you perform
better too.

EXERCISE: THE SAFE WAY TO

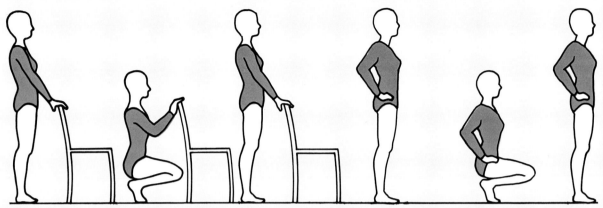

Most people know they need more exercise but are not sure how to get it. They may try a keep-fit routine for a few days, a quick jog round the local park, or perhaps a swim on a Sunday morning. But because they have no exercise plan or objective it is easy to give up keep fit resolutions. Yet regular exercise is vital to health and helps improve the way you look and feel and establishes good eating and sleeping patterns. Without it the muscles waste and atrophy, become listless, and we die younger. Like successful dieting, successful exercise is a matter of changing your habits and incorporating new activities into your lifestyle. The first few weeks and months may be difficult and require patience and some courage – old habits really do die hard – but exercise can become an **enjoyable** new habit surprisingly quickly. This chapter shows how to approach exercise so that you achieve this goal. We assume that most people are relatively unfit and have lost some of the natural confidence and joy in using their bodies they probably felt as children or teenagers. They need now to explore exercise as if it were a lost continent to find which kind or routine suits them best. Some people thrive on a regular series of exercises, some like running, some swear by yoga (a form of physical **and** mental exercise) while others go in for squash or swimming. Because no one method is right for everyone, you need to keep an open mind about which might suit you, and be prepared to discard some and try others. You need, too, to experiment with **when** to exercise and **how much**. We begin with a series of simple exercise routines for which you need no equipment and hardly any space, based on work by former

British Olympic Coaching Advisor Alistair Murray now Director of London's City Gym Health Clinic, for the Health Education Council. Unlike most published exercise routines they are designed for the **average** person who wants to be fit rather than for a super athlete. Do them for eight weeks or so and they will help to bring the joy of exercise back into your life.

THE RIGHT WAY TO EXERCISE

The big danger when you start a programme of exercise is that you may try to do too much too soon. As a result you may give up soon after starting, discouraged by the discovery that you are not as fit as you had hoped and by the very real effort that you find is involved. Another result is that you may cause yourself harm – by straining either leg, arm or back muscles which are unused to sudden heavier activity, or your heart muscle. Such dangers are very real and anyone over the age of thirty-five starting an exercise programme should have a full check-up with a doctor first – and a discussion too if the doctor is sympathetic. Anyone **under** thirty-five who has any doubts at all about his or her fitness to exercise should also see a doctor. It is for these reasons that our exercise programme, based on the work of Alistair Murray, one of Britain's most experienced physical trainers and a specialist in the training (re-training is a better word) of the unfit, takes things **slowly and pleasantly**. The object is to enjoy yourself from Day one, not to drop out exhausted and aching on Day three.

START

YOUR PULSE RATE

You can start our programme right now by sitting down and taking your own pulse. This is easily done by turning the palm of one hand towards the ceiling and placing the first three fingers of the other just above the point where the thumb joins the wrist. It may take a moment or two actually to feel the beat of the pulse but you will soon get used to it. Now count the beats on a wrist watch for 60 seconds and you will have your pulse rate. Your pulse shows the speed at which your heart beats as it circulates blood around your body. The heart rate itself reflects the oxygen content of the blood – the lower the content the more the heart hurries to supply the body with oxygen-carrying blood. This is why your heart and pulse rate rise when you run, or indeed when you are stressed, to supply the body with the extra oxygen it needs to cope with the new demand made upon it. Actual pulse rates vary widely and so in themselves are no great indication of health or ill-health. But men have an average pulse rate between 70 and 75 beats in a minute, and 80 to 85 as boys. Women have higher average rates – 75 to 80 beats a minute as women, around 85 as girls. But these are **average** figures and it is possible to be in normal good health with a resting pulse as low as 50 or as high as 100.

What is more important to you personally is how your pulse rate changes with activity and exercise. In an unfit person a pulse **tends** to be weak, a little irregular, faster, and to rise more quickly with exertion. With more regular exercise the opposite trends occur:
– The pulse gets stronger
– It gets 'bigger' because the artery expands
– It becomes more regular
– Its frequency drops
– It becomes harder to raise it to a particular point by exertion.
– It recovers to its 'normal' rate faster.

SAFE EXERCISE

From this you can see that you can use your pulse rate to increase your exercise at a safe rate which your body can put up with. For if you can work out what your own maximum 'safe' pulse rate is, then you know you are exercising safely if you keep it to this level. At the same time you can deduce that the more you exercise the harder it will become to raise it to the maximum level, and in this way you have a way of checking that you are getting fitter **safely**. There is a simple rule of thumb, now accepted as medically safe by the British Health Education Council, by which you can establish your own maximum 'safe' pulse rate. All you do is to subtract your age from 200 and then subtract a further 40 handicap if you are unfit. On this basis a woman of forty would have a personal safe pulse level of 120:

	200
less age	40
	———
	160
less fitness factor	40
	———
	120

As fitness improves you can reduce your handicap until it disappears. If you are over forty-five it is wise to keep a handicap of between ten and twenty. It should be stressed that this **is** a rule of thumb so that if you exceed your pulse level you will not immediately collapse. indeed very few people cause themselves permanent harm by exercise – but because the risk is there we believe it is not worth anyone's while taking it. Armed with a way of measuring your exercise level so that you stay within very safe limits, what do you do with it? In the heart and lung exercises that follow – and this also includes popular keep-fit methods like jogging and squash – the aim is to maintain the maximum 'safe' pulse rate for a period of ten minutes continuous exercise. At first, as we have said, your pulse will race up to the maximum level very quickly and you will have to take frequent rests to keep it within its limits. Later these rest periods become less frequent until you can go through a whole ten minutes of continuous exercise without bringing the pulse rate above the maximum level.

At first this method of checking your progress may seem irksome and confusing, but you will quickly find it has a very useful purpose. For if you keep a record of your pulse rate after each exercise routine (in the heart and lung group of exercises) you will find yourself encouraged by your own progress. It may not progress regularly but it **will** progress and seeing it do so is a very real encouragement to keep going. Also, whatever the aches and pains you suffer in the early days, you know you will be exercising in a safe way. Though it is worth re-emphasising that if you are over thirty-five, have any doubt about exercising whatever your age, or are under any kind of medication (which may affect your pulse rate) or over-weight, you should see your doctor.

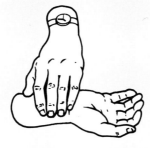

BEFORE STARTING

– Learn how to take your pulse
– Work out your maximum safe pulse rate
– Keep a regular record of your pulse rate
– and enjoy your exercise in the knowledge that you are starting it in a safe (if sometimes slow) way.

STANDARD SCHEDULE 1

By now you should want to incorporate some kind of regular exercise into your lifestyle. The best way to start is **slowly** and **safely** and the enjoyable routines outlined in the next six pages are designed with those needs in mind.

It is likely that you have exercised so little in the last few months or years that you may be discouraged or too easily injured if you rush into a violent sport or a punishing routine of keep-fit exercises. It is because of this risk that Alistair Murray, when he first designed exercise routines for the British Health Education Council, divided them into two categories – the Standard Schedule for the average unfit person who wants to start exercising again; and the Advanced Schedule for the reasonably fit who wants something more demanding. Make sure first that you can do all the exercises in the Standard Schedule comfortably and with no strain. The schedules use three different kinds of exercise, each designed to cater for a different facet of your exercise needs.

MOBILITY EXERCISES make sure that all the main joints and muscles are taken through their complete range of movement.

STRENGTHENING EXERCISES slowly build up your capacity to cope with sudden and unusual physical demands that may be made on you. It is very easy for the unfit to pull muscles or strain backs doing 'normal' things like lifting a heavy weight in the garden at the weekend, going on a long country walk, or running for a bus. You can build up the strength needed for such contingencies by exercising regularly against some form of resistance, and these exercises help you achieve this.

HEART AND LUNG EXERCISES strengthen a muscle that many people forget they have – the heart. They also help create steadier and deeper breathing habits which appear to have such an important role in helping us to combat stress. To achieve this we increase the body's demand for oxygen, mainly by exercising the major muscle groups of legs, arms and trunk. Once you get used to doing the exercises you will be able to complete them in about fifteen minutes, perhaps three times a week.

For most people it seems to work better if they do them at a regular time of day – before breakfast and before the evening meal are two favoured periods. Also try to get into a routine of doing them on specific days – there are times when one doesn't feel like doing them, or there doesn't seem to be time, and a schedule helps get over this problem. You will find it best to have special clothes for your exercise periods – shorts and singlet is adequate for men and leotard with tights without feet (giving greater mobility) for women.

When you exercise you celebrate the fact that you can exercise – so do it slowly and peacefully, even if it **does** sometimes leave you panting.

These five mobility exercises should be done slowly in a relaxed tempo. Never force or push yourself – an increase in range will come in its own time. Do ten to twelve repetitions of each movement and do not increase the number, or the speed at which you do them. Progress comes from increasing the range of movement and then maintaining a new level of flexibility as you reach it.

1 ARM SWINGING
Position: Feet wide apart, arms hanging loosely by your sides.
Movement: Raise both arms together, forward, upwards, backwards and sideways in a circular motion, brushing your ears with your arms as they go past.

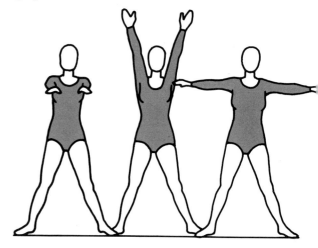

2 SIDE BENDS

Position: Feet wide apart, hands on hips.
Movement: Keeping the head at right angles to the trunk, bend at the hips first to the left, then to the right.

3 TRUNK, KNEE AND HIP BENDS

Position: Stand 18 inches behind the back of a chair with hands resting lightly on the back.
Movement: Raise the left knee and bring the forehead down to meet it. Repeat with the right knee. The movement should be long and strong – do not rush or do it jerkily. Eventually you can dispense with the chair, working from a standing position with the supporting leg slightly bent.

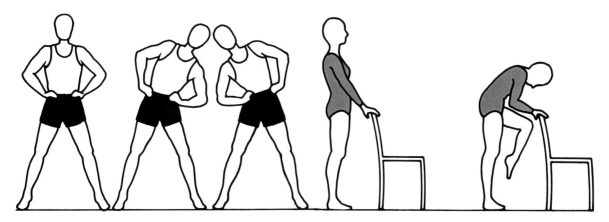

4 HEAD, ARMS AND TRUNK ROTATING

Position: Feet wide apart, hands and arms reaching directly forwards at shoulder level.
Movement: Turn the head, arms and shoulders around to the left as far as you can go **without strain,** bending the right arm across the chest; then repeat the movement to the right. Keep the hips and legs still throughout.

5 ALTERNATE ANKLE REACH

Position: Feet wide apart, both palms on the front of the upper left thigh.
Movement: Relax the trunk forward as you slide both hands down the front of the left leg.
Return to upright position then repeat to the right.
IF YOU SUFFER EVEN MILD BACK TROUBLE DO NOT PASS THE KNEES WITH THE HANDS.

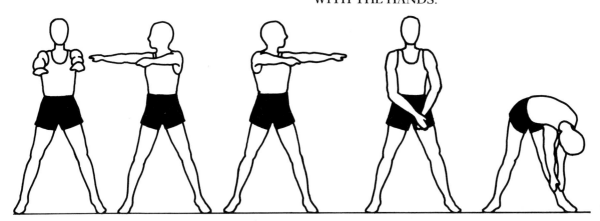

STANDARD SCHEDULE 2

STRENGTH EXERCISES

These consist of three groups of exercises: press-ups, for the chest, arm and shoulder muscles; abdominal exercises; and leg exercises. Each group is broken down into four stages because unfit people may easily strain themselves if they start doing the full exercise too rigorously. The traditional press-up, for example, is too strenuous for unfit or overweight people. Start at the lowest level of each exercise with about ten repetitions. Progress slowly until you can do twenty-five repetitions comfortably and only then go on to the next level for that exercise.

PRESS-UPS

Level One: Stand facing a wall so that, with your arms outstretched, you can just touch it with your palms. Stand on your toes and then bend the arms so that your chest and chin touch the wall. Return to starting position by straightening arms, keeping the body straight throughout.

Level Two: Again standing, place the hands about a foot apart on a **secure** table or flat surface. Bend arms, keeping body straight until chest touches the table and then return to start position. WOMEN NEED NOT PROGRESS BEYOND THIS STAGE.

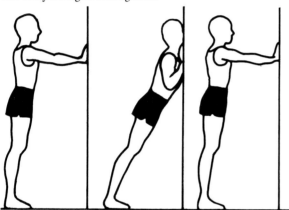
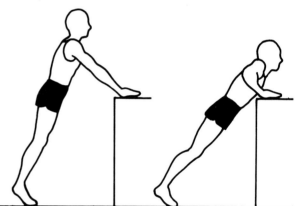

Level Three: The same as level two but using a chair or stool. Be sure the chair is steady and your head can clear the back as you go down.

Level Four: When you can do twenty-five repetitions at level three you are ready for full press-ups. Place the hands on the floor directly under the shoulders with the fingers pointing forward. Chest and chin touch the floor, arms straighten, hold, and then lower again. Do the exercise at a steady pace, neither fast nor too slow.

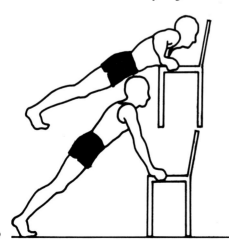
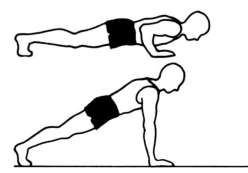

ABDOMINAL EXERCISES

These exercises, which help flatten your stomach muscles, are very helpful BUT MUST NOT BE HURRIED. Take each level as it comes, working up progressively to about twenty-five repetitions, before moving on.

REMEMBER ALISTAIR MURRAY'S ADVICE: 'Heroics are not only silly, they can be dangerous. Do not be in a hurry to progress.'

Level One: Sit on the front part of a secure chair, legs straight and heels on floor. Lean back and grip the side of the seat for support. Bend the knees and bring the fronts of the thighs up to squeeze gently against the body. For most people this may be difficult to do at first, so take it easily.

Level Two: Do the same exercise but with the legs held straight.

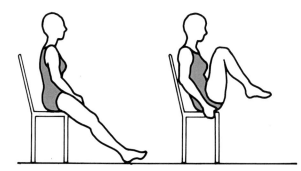

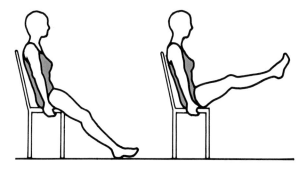

Level Three: Lie on your back, knees slightly bent, with your feet tucked under a heavy chair or settee. Arms stretched back behind you. Swing up to a sitting position but do not stretch any further forward than hands on ankles.

Level Four: Lie on your back with your hands cupped behind your head and your heels on the edge of a chair. Swing up to a sitting position, letting your knees bend slightly as you do so.

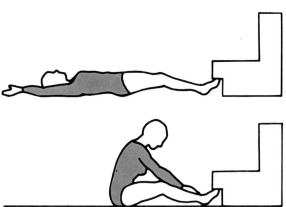

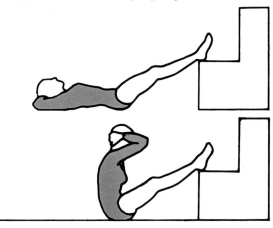

STANDARD SCHEDULE 3

LEG EXERCISES

If you sink from a standing position to a squat and up again more than a few times you may quickly become aware of a weakness in the legs. These exercises use squats as a way of strengthening your leg muscles.

Level One: Stand 18 inches behind a chair with your hands on the back. Lower the body into a squat keeping the feet flat on the floor. Straighten both legs and come up on the toes, then return to a vertical position again.

Level Two: The same as level one but without the chair and with the hands on the hips.

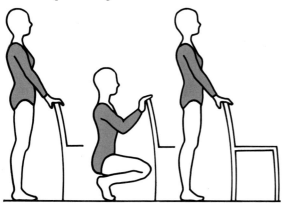

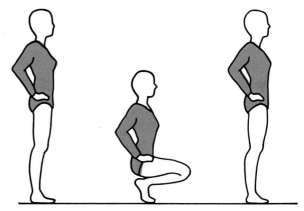

Level Three: The same as level two but come up from the squat fast so that your feet actually leave the floor, at first only a few inches, then a bit higher.

Level Four: Start in the half squat illustrated and leap upwards with arms and leg outstretching into a star shape. As you land bring the feet together and give at the knees to take the shock.
Again, remember, DO NOT BE IN A HURRY TO PROGRESS.

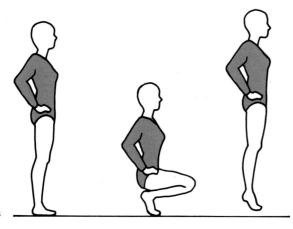

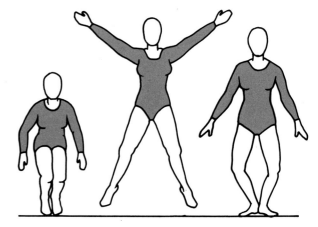

HEART AND LUNG EXERCISES

Your pulse rate tells you how hard the heart muscle is being exercised, so check page 77 on how to monitor your pulse. Check your pulse rate frequently when doing the heart and lung exercises, especially in the first few weeks.

Level One: Running on the spot: Simply stand with your arms loosely by your side and gently run on the spot. Do not begin by raising the knees high, but aim to get them higher as you progress. It is helpful to have a watch or clock with a second hand placed somewhere easy to read so that you can time yourself comfortably. Start by running on the spot for only thirty seconds and gradually build up to six minutes, **constantly** checking your pulse to see that it is within your maximum safe level. Remember that at first you will have to stop frequently to keep it within the maximum level and then, as you get faster, your activity periods will get longer before the pulse rises to the maximum level.

Level Two: Bench stepping: For this exercise find a stable box or stool which can take your weight. Stand 12 inches away from it with hands on hips. Step up fifteen times on to it with the left foot leading, and then fifteen times with the right foot leading. Increase by one step per foot each session until you reach a maximum of thirty steps with each foot. Then gradually raise the height you are stepping up to a maximum of 18 inches. Once you can bench step to this height comfortably start working up to a continuous stepping programme until you can do six minutes without a break **within your maximum safe pulse level.**

Level Three: Outdoor exercise: Few of us have rooms big enough to use as gymnasia, so as you progress with your exercise you will want to move outdoors. Choose between jogging, swimming and cycling and aim to do ten minutes continuously. Swimming is one of the best all-round activities there is, but climate or circumstance may make this hard for you to do. Cycling also has limitations – it **is** a dangerous activity in a normal urban situation, as accident figures sadly show. Drivers are largely unaware of cyclists' needs and limitations, and often do not seem to 'see' them. For this reason it is necessary to cycle defensively – always being one step ahead of any possible hazard – and this does not make for relaxed exercise. However, if you can find somewhere really safe to cycle – a park, or in the country – it is an ideal exercise, and one you can grade to your needs. For these reasons we believe that jogging has most advantages for most people as a method of regular activity to fit into our programme and we show on pages 88–89 how to approach it to get the best from it.

FINALLY – remember to exercise in a relaxed way and with pleasure. Three sessions a week of up to 20 minutes each are enough, especially in the early stages. Monitor your progress and expect to move ahead quickly at some stages, and slowly at others. Experiment with the time of day when you exercise, and with the range of activities you do.

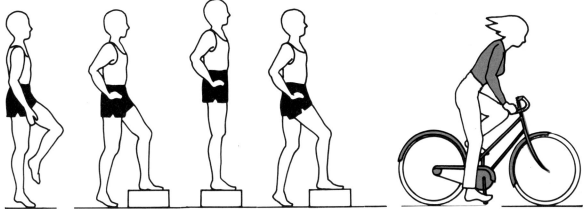

ADVANCED SCHEDULE 1

The Advanced Schedule, devised by former British Olympic Coaching Advisor Alistair Murray, is for those who are already fit and want to get fitter. Only those who have comfortably completed the basic schedule should attempt it and once again the emphasis is on doing the exercises slowly and safely. Their appeal for the average person is that they can be done at home without special equipment. However, since the exercises use weights to increase the effort needed to go through them it may pay you to invest in a bar-bell and a dumb-bell. These are relatively cheap for the benefits they give you, and are easier to hold and increase in weight than improvised equipment.

If you do want to improvise then the easiest method is to fill two plastic washing-up liquid containers with water (or sand) and use these instead. Different sizes will naturally give you different weights but the average size weighs 2 pounds filled with water (double, filled with sand). Fill them **full** otherwise the water or sand tends to shift, which may upset your rhythm and balance doing the exercises. In the diagrams we show a bar-bell being used, although you can substitute two hand dumb-bells instead. But buy the proper equipment if you can.

HOW TO APPROACH THE SCHEDULE

Begin each session with the mobility exercises outlined in the basic schedule.

This warming-up period is important and should not be skipped.

There are ten exercises in the Advanced Schedule and they should be done successively each exercise session. Begin by doing only eight to ten repetitions of each and then build up to a maximum of thirty each in each session. As before, take reasonable rests between each session and check your pulse rate as you go along, keeping it within the maximum level.

As your stamina improves you will be able to do more repetitions of each exercise and reduce the rest periods.

Again, **never strain, never try heroics.** This programme is not a ten-minute competition to show that you are better than someone else but a change in lifestyle to take you towards better health. For this reason you should aim to enjoy every session and not worry about your progress. This will come in its own time – and probably a lot faster if you don't rush it!

EQUIPMENT TO USE

Weight training equipment can easily be improvised at home if you do not want to buy any. It must always be secure and stable – so if you use plastic bottles (NEVER glass) filled with water or sand ensure they are sealed and quite full. Keep all equipment (especially heavier bar-bells and dumb-bells) away from children. A sturdy, heavy training mat is useful and remember to train well clear of doors and windows to avoid accidents.

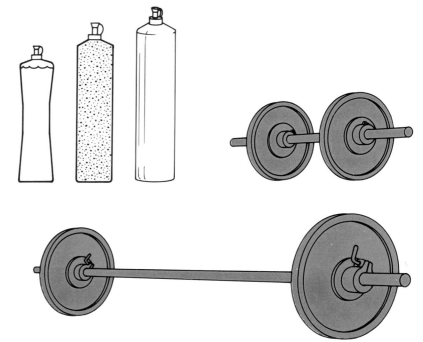

1 CHIN HIGH PULL

Toes beneath the bar about 10 inches apart. Bend knees, looking straight to the front and keeping the back flat but not vertical. Grip the bar with the knuckles towards the front. Stand upright, pulling the bar vertically close to the body until it is under your chin. Complete the movement by lowering the bar to the thighs and then bending the legs back to the starting position.

2 PALMS FORWARD CURL

Stand erect, holding the bar down at arm's length against the body at the top of the thighs. Flex the arms to bring the bar up to the chest and then return to the starting position. Keep the rest of the body still throughout.

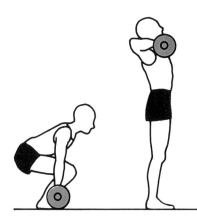

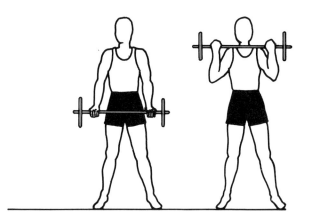

3 PRESS BEHIND BACK

Stand erect with the bar resting across the back of the neck. Extend arms to full length above the head and return to starting position.

4 'ROWING'

Bend forward in rowing position at 45 degrees with the feet well apart. The bar-bell hangs vertically above the ground with knuckles facing forward. Raise the bar until it touches the top of your chest. Keep the rest of the body still. **Repeat no more than fifteen times.**

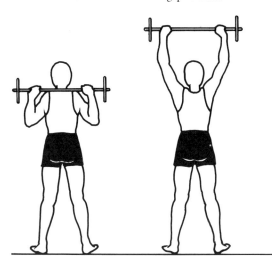

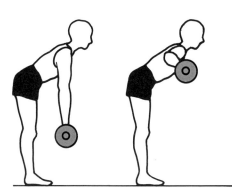

ADVANCED SCHEDULE 2

5 SIDE BENDS

With feet well apart hold dumb-bell in your left hand, with the right hand on hip. Bend to the left as far as you can without strain and then to the right. The dumb-bell hangs loosely throughout. Do your repetitions on one side first and then change hands and repeat on the other. Do not keep changing the dumb-bell from one side to another.

6 SQUATS

With feet about 10 inches apart place bar-bell behind back supported by hands. Bend knees, keeping back straight until the thighs are almost parallel then come up briskly on tiptoe. Lower back to starting position with feet flat on the floor.

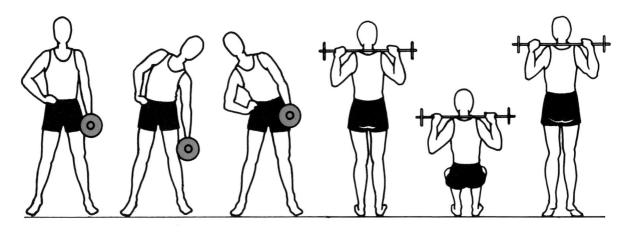

7 BENCH PRESS

Lie on your back on a firm bench, with knees flexed (a table will do if you have no bench but make sure it is firm, and easy to climb onto). Bar-bell rests on chest with palms forward. Extend arms to full length and lower again.

8 CLEAN AND PRESS

Start in the same position as exercise 1. Extend body and pull bar straight up close to the body until it rests on top of the chest. Press bar overhead to arm's length. Lower bar to chest and then thighs and bend legs and lower into starting position.

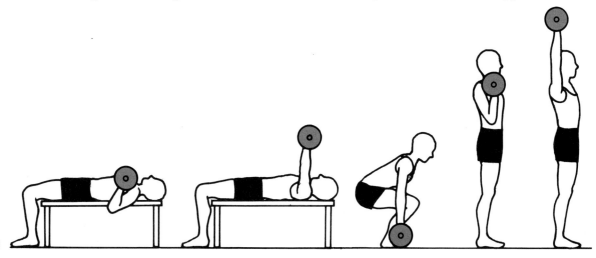

9 SIT-UPS

There are no weights in this exercise, but it adds balance to the schedule at this point. Go back to the sit-ups described in level four of the abdominal exercises in the basic schedule and make sure you can do twenty-five repetitions comfortably. Now lie on back with arms outstretched on the ground behind the head. Raise legs, trunk and arms simultaneously as if trying to grasp ankles with the hands. Return to lying position.

REMEMBER: DO ALL THESE EXERCISES SLOWLY AND SAFELY AND DO NOT BE IN A HURRY TO PROGRESS. BEGIN EACH SESSION WITH A QUIET MOMENT OR TWO. GIVE YOURSELF PLENTY OF TIME FOR THE SESSION.

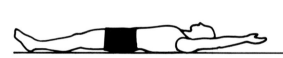
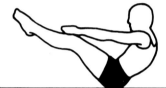

10 STRAIGHT ARM PULL-OVER

This 'quietening-down' exercise concludes each session and you should use a very light weight because more leverage is involved than in the other exercises. Lie on your back on the bench or table with bar across the thighs, palms downwards. Raise bar back in an arc to behind the head and then return to the resting position, keeping the arms straight throughout.

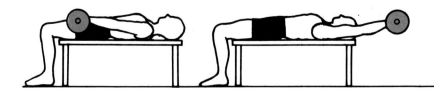

JOGGING

Jogging is an increasingly popular form of exercise and relaxation because it is simple to organise and is fun. But because it is easy to start the wrong way many people stop jogging after only a week or two, or do it too infrequently for it to be much use. These two pages show how to approach jogging, how to find out if it suits your particular needs, and the best ways to integrate it into a healthy lifestyle.

WHAT JOGGING DOES FOR YOU
Jogging stimulates the cardiovascular system and helps reduce the level of cholesterol in the blood. The rapid improvement many people show in stamina and general well being after starting regular jogging suggests that it is good for health. Among many it appears to reduce stress tension and increase mental balance and peace – though this is more an impression given by joggers, who report that they attain states of peace and euphoria similar to those resulting from some form of meditation or meditative exercise like yoga. Equally, however, many people find it a hard slog which they can never get used to however slowly they start. This is a form of regular exercise to try with an open mind, and give up in favour of something else if (after a reasonable trial) it does not suit you or your circumstances.

BEFORE YOU START . . .
Remember that jogging should be fun, not a form of self-inflicted torture. It is not necessary to gasp and pant mile after mile to make jogging a healthy exercise. In fact, just the opposite. Our warning to take it easy at the start applies to jogging as to other forms of new exercise. Remember that jogging is a creative exercise, or should be. Too many joggers, even regular ones, run the same route day after day in the same way. This is like taking an identical holiday year after year, or shopping in the same shop all the time. It gets boring and loses some of the contribution to your health that it can make. Finally, try from the outset to be non-competitive about it. Do not set out to compare the speed or distance you run with other people you know who go jogging. Later you may want to test your ability by timing yourself over distances but first your sole aim should be to enjoy the freedom and grace of running at your own speed in your own way, over your own route.

WHAT TO WEAR
The most important piece of equipment you need is a good pair of running shoes. Because so many urban-based joggers must run on hard surfaces part or all of the time, it is essential to get shoes that are well cushioned and give good heel support. You risk damaging your feet otherwise. However, running shoes to suit **you** are often hard to find, so do not expect to buy them from the first sports shops you visit. Always try both shoes on, and keep them on for several minutes, walking, jumping, standing on tiptoes and generally trying them out for feel. When you buy them get some cotton-based running socks as well – some have a slightly padded heel and sole which is comfortable. Many women will find it more comfortable to wear a bra when jogging – it can also help stop chafing of nipples, which can be a problem.
The best thing to wear on the rest of you is a tracksuit – preferably a cotton-based one because it will be cooler in warm weather and warmer in cold weather than synthetic fibres.

ENJOY YOURSELF
Jogging should never ever be a slog, so set out to enjoy it from the start. Begin by walking a hundred yards or so, giving yourself time to take some deep breaths of fresh air, and stretch your arms above your head. Then start slowly looking around and taking in the scene: if it's a nice morning take pleasure in it . . . if it's nasty, well, at least you are doing something about it. If you begin to get a little puffed, stop and do some knee-bends. Walk a bit more. Do some standing press-ups against a tree or wall; leave the full press-ups till later. As you jog try jumping and stretching upwards, or hopping or taking bigger strides for a few paces. Make it interesting for yourself and use as much of your body as you can.

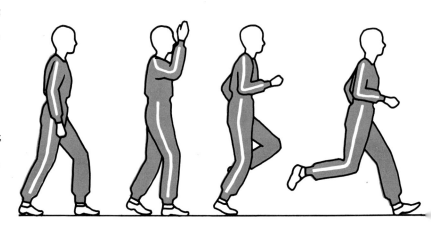

WHEN SHALL I JOG?

There is no best time for everyone, though one of two daily periods seem best – early in the morning before breakfast or in the early evening before the final meal of the day. On balance the early evening seems to suit more people – it fits in with work schedules better and many find they are more physically awake then.

REMEMBER . . . do our initial programme of exercises before you start regular jogging if you are unfit, or have not exercised regularly for a long time. Use the safe pulse-check method of monitoring your progress outlined on page 77. And don't jog if you feel unwell or are recovering from a cold or 'flu.

THE FIRST FEW DAYS

If you are reluctant to get started remember that almost every jogger you see has faced the same problem. However, it may help to take our advice and start your daily jog by **walking**. There is a real difference between ten minutes' steady walking, with nothing but exercise in mind, and the average scurry-and-slouch-with-a-purpose that many of us adopt. Try it and see. Put on your running shoes and tracksuit and simply walk for ten to fifteen minutes daily for four or five days. Enjoy the freedom from pressure involved in doing **nothing** but walking. This may not be what you expect exercise to feel like but it is exercise, and it will prepare you for your first jogging sessions. When you start jogging do it for very short periods of less than a minute each time (unless you are already reasonably fit). Jog for a short period at a reasonable pace and then walk for a little. Then jog again, and so on.

A **reasonable** pace is one that leaves you with enough breath to talk comfortably if there is someone with you. You should feel only slightly breathless at the end of these initial sessions – if you feel fatigued you are trying too hard, so slow down. Do about two weeks of this very light jogging, interspersed with longer periods of walking. In this time you will begin to learn to feel the rhythm of running and the satisfaction in keeping it up for long enough to feel you have exerted yourself. After two or three weeks start extending the jogging periods, but keep the total jog/walk session within fifteen minutes altogether. You may be tempted to push yourself, but resist the temptation. You will be making much more progress that you think, and you will be enjoying it. After four to six weeks the average jogger is able to keep going at a **reasonable** pace for five minutes or so, perhaps a little longer. A good target is to try to keep going at a pace at which you can still jog and talk for ten minutes – and this may take up to ten weeks or so, depending on your initial condition. Once you can jog steadily for ten minutes you are on your own – able to enjoy developing your approach to this most flexible of regular exercises. The only two rules you need keep in mind are to try to do it regularly and to aim always to enjoy it. And try to run in a relaxed way – do not run stiffly or with hunched, tense shoulders.

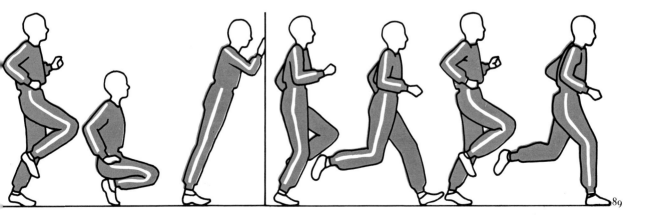

YOGA

Yoga is a system of physical and mental exercises from the East which is being slowly tried and adopted in the West. Like any great philosophy or way of life, it has taken centuries to develop and is the result of collective thinking and wisdom of doctor-monks and students of yoga. For this reason yoga is not something you can learn quickly or from a book, like typing or French. Yet some of its techniques – particularly the physical postures and routines from Hatha Yoga (a branch of yoga concerned with mastering the physical body) – can be fairly easily learned and benefited from by almost anyone.

We have included these two pages on yoga in this section because most Westerners' introduction to it will be via Hatha Yoga, the most physical form of yoga. The six 'exercises' – they are really postures or asanas – on these pages should be regarded as merely a taste of something which is best learnt from a trained instructor on a yoga course.

If you perform these routines daily over a period of two or three weeks you may be surprised at the calming physical and mental affects they can have. But we stress: yoga is best learnt personally from an instructor, so this is **only** a brief introduction. Wear clothes which do not restrict movement and which keep you warm. Choose a quiet, uncluttered place to do the routines, insist on not being disturbed (and some people use the same mat or towel each time for the asanas to help them concentrate). Do not do them after a main meal and relax for two minutes before starting.

To start with, you should hold each posture for ten seconds. As you progress you can hold it for longer but never strain to do so. Yoga is not competitive. If you do feel strain then you are overdoing things – give your muscles time to adapt to the demands you are making on them, in their own time.

At the end of the session lie down in the relaxed position on the floor and untense your whole body – starting from the toes and working upwards. This is the yoga nidra – deep relaxation. When your whole body is relaxed focus your mind on something soothing and pleasurable. Take about ten minutes over this and, at the end, get up slowly and calmly.

ASANA ONE: stretch

Stand straight, arms by sides. Slowly raise arms above head until palms touch. Slowly stand on tiptoe. Hold for ten seconds, breathing regularly through the nose – not your mouth. Lower heels to floor. Bring hands slowly back to sides. Stand still for a few seconds. Repeat three times.

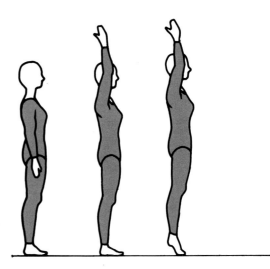

ASANA FOUR: alternate kneebends

Lying on the floor, bring your right knee up towards you, clasping it with both hands. Raise your head to meet your knee – hold for a few seconds. Slowly relax down again. Do this three times with the right knee, three times with the left. Then relax for ten seconds.

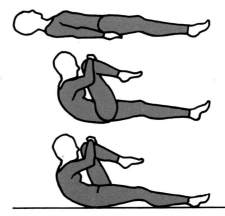

ASANA TWO: swing

Stand with feet as wide apart as possible, body straight, hands by sides. Bring arms above head, palms together. Swing out to the right with arms and sweep down to the floor and round and up again. Do this three times and then repeat in opposite direction.

Before starting the next asana, relax on the floor for ten seconds.

ASANA THREE: side slip

Kneel, resting back on your heels. Raise your hands above your head with palms meeting. Without moving your legs, slide your body over to the right; hold for ten seconds. Repeat twice. Do the same on the left side.

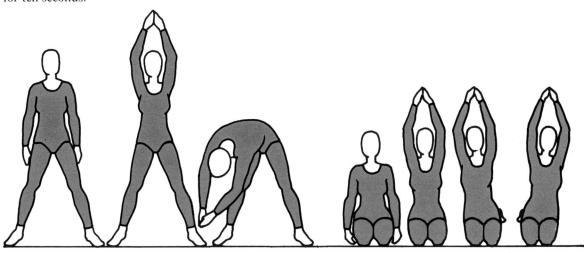

ASANA FIVE: leg raising (1)

Lying on your back, raise your right leg up straight – as near right angles to your body as you can. Hold for ten seconds. Repeat. Do the same with the left leg.

ASANA SIX: leg raising (2)

Lying flat on the floor place both legs together. Raise them up straight and lower them seven times in a smooth, uninterrupted rhythm. On the seventh time, as you bring them down, halt about a foot from the floor and hold for ten seconds.

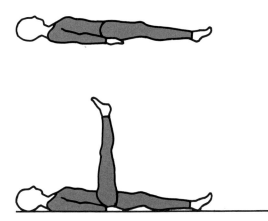

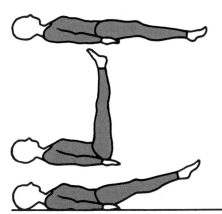

SWIMMING, WALKING....

These pages show how to approach three popular sports which need only a little equipment or training and which all the family can enjoy: swimming, cycling and walking. As with jogging, however, you need to know what you are doing to get the most out of them, and you need to be persistent in the first two or three weeks of starting them to get into the routines and acquire the special skills (not difficult) each of them demands.

SWIMMING

Swimming gives your body better all-round exercise than any other sport. A combination of crawl, back- and breast-strokes for fifteen minutes a day will put you through a full range of strengthening, mobility and heart and lung exercises. Like all good exercise swimming is also very relaxing – perhaps it is the fact of changing and putting yourself into a different element and the invigorating rub-down afterwards that make it so revitalising. It has the major advantage for a family that it is something everyone can do together and because it is a physical contact sport it is one way of breaking down barriers. No wonder so many fathers, who may see little of their family during the week, like to take their children swimming at the weekend. But to get the most out of it you need to plan carefully what you are actually going to do when you are in the water. Treading water talking to family and friends is not exercise; nor is swimming one quick length and then floating on your back for the rest of the time. Remember the basic aim of exercise for health is to raise your pulse to your 'exercise' level (see page 77) and **keep it there** for a reasonable time. Also, you need to exercise yourself fully by combining the three elements stressed in our basic fitness schedule – mobility, heart and lung strength. You get these elements, and much needed variety, by going through a routine of

five minutes of breaststroke, five of the crawl and five of backstroke. Simple and effective. But if you have not swum for a long time, or are just starting to exercise again, this will be too much. We suggest therefore that you start with two minutes of each (six minutes total) with two minutes' rest between (floating, treading water, or chatting to friends by the side of the pool). This makes a total of ten minutes in all to start with, after which you can build up to a continuous routine of up to fifteen minutes as with our fitness schedules. The ability of individuals to stay in the water without getting cold varies very widely indeed, so trust no-one's instinct but your own. Fifteen minutes is a good average, but many find ten minutes enough. This is sufficient time to get all the exercise you need, so if you get cold easily do not turn the whole thing into an endurance test by staying in too long.

One problem with weekend swimming in crowded pools is that there simply isn't space to get a good rhythm going, or to swim continuously in the way you will eventually want to. So try an early morning swim (many public pools open early for this purpose) or try reorganising your schedule so you can get to a pool when it is uncrowded. If you can manage a swim every day, that's ideal, but few can. Three sessions a week of fifteen minutes each is a good target, and will help maintain your fitness or build it up.

WALKING

Hard rambling and hill walking can be real exercise because they can stretch you physically and mentally. Their disadvantage is that they take a lot of time relative to other sports and the right locations may not be available to you. Most holidays can easily include these kinds of heavy walking, and they can be fitted in for at least some weekends each year as well. This may seem a long way from a regular programme of exercises, of a daily swim or jog, but better health comes about by using the body and mind in a full range of activities and situations – and rough walking is one of the best. It is worth taking time to get the right equipment – principally boots which support the ankles, a well-designed anorak, and warm trousers (avoid shorts), large-scale maps and compass. Also consider taking advantage of one of the many courses (often subsidised) available to teach the skills of hill walking, map-work, how to use a compass (a surprising number of people carrying them do not know how to use them), and how to survive in difficult conditions.

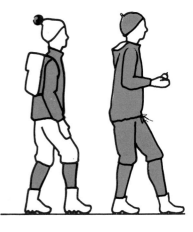

AND CYCLING

SAFETY Every year people suffer injury and fatality from not knowing how to handle the risks involved in swimming, cycling and hill walking. It is well worth the time and trouble involved for any individual starting these activities to take one of the widely available basic courses designed to show them how to follow their interest safely. Local public swimming pools will usually organise courses in life saving; while cycling courses are now widely available and **very** worthwhile. Hill walking and survival courses are more expensive but taken as a form of holiday are a good investment. It is worth putting all children through such courses because of the basic skills they teach, the self-reliance and confidence they encourage, and the value they will have to others in years ahead. A very good investment for long-term health!

CYCLING

Like swimming, cycling can be a complete exercise. As well as using the legs, feet and ankles, it involves the arms, shoulders, back, and abdominal and diaphragmatic muscles. On top of this, it is mentally stimulating. Its major disadvantage is that for city dwellers there are few places to cycle without competing with cars, pedestrians and polluted air. And in traffic-ridden major cities it is dangerous enough to be a stressful activity, and we do not recommend it for exercise. City-bound people **can** buy a cycle exercise machine, but it is a relatively big investment for something you can get free by taking up another activity like jogging and swimming. Elsewhere, cycling is such good exercise that it is worth incorporating into your lifestyle.

BUYING A BICYCLE

Like a good suit of clothes, a bicycle should fit you. The key measurement is the distance between the centre of the saddle (**1**) and the bottom bracket, the tube in which the pedals revolve (**2**). This should be the distance between your pubic bone and the floor (measured in stockinged feet) **less** 9 inches; or your height divided by three. Either way you should be able to sit on the saddle with your feet just flat on the ground. The nose of the saddle (**3**) should be about 2 inches behind a vertical line through the bottom bracket. The handle part of the handle-bars (**4**) should be set at 10 degrees from the vertical, the lower end towards you. This is for drop handlebars, which are the best kind to have for exercise cycling. They give more balance and the freedom to push harder. However, for town and city cycling drop handlebars are less manageable for inexperienced cyclists, and they may be positively harmful for back-pain sufferers. So for learner cyclists upright handlebars are often better. Gears are essential – they allow you to maintain the same level of effort at different speeds – but traditional three-speed gears are inadequate for most cyclists. Five- or ten-speed gears are best, with preference for the more manageable five-speed gears for all but the really experienced. Before buying take a lot of advice, preferably at a specialist shop with a good stock. Wheel size sometimes worries cycle buyers because, while small wheels are popular, the experts mainly use bigger wheels. Our advice is to follow the experts – bigger wheels also tend to be more stable. Toe clips make for easier pedalling and encourage you to pedal in the correct way. This is to push with the ball of your foot on your pedal, using the ankle to power the pedal.

As with other sports, the best way to build up cycling as a form of exercise is slowly and steadily. But for most people cycling will be not a main sport but an exercise well worth incorporating into daily living.

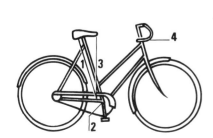

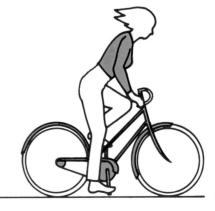

EAT FOR PLEASURE AND HEALTH

The ideal diet is one that gives you a healthy, vigorous life and prevents deficiencies. The best way to achieve this, day by day, is to understand the food your body needs, and why.

There are people who follow good diets out of habit – but many have strayed from the path over the years and have included in their diet a lot of things that are simply not really necessary, and that taken in quantity can be positively harmful.

If you are only just beginning to appreciate how much health depends on the food you eat then initially it is going to need a conscious daily effort to establish a new, healthier eating pattern.

Look at the groups of foods below. Now make a list of all the foods you normally eat in the course of a day and ring round those not included in the food groups – there will probably be several!

Ask yourself if it was really necessary to have that bar of chocolate mid-morning, that heavy sweet course at lunch or those extra cups of coffee.

If you start by being really critical of yourself – and there is no one else who will help you so well – then you will find your food habits will change naturally.

The foods that are essential to health and form the basis of a good, balanced diet come from four main groups.

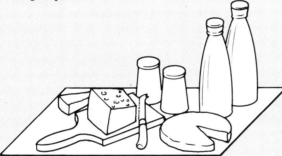

MILK GROUP
Includes milk, yogurt, cheese and provides protein, fat, carbohydrates, calcium and vitamin A.

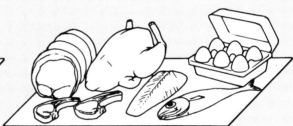

MEAT GROUP
Includes all meats, poultry, fish and eggs and provides protein, fat, iron, Vitamin B and Vitamins A and D.

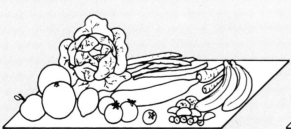

VEGETABLE AND FRUIT GROUP
Includes green vegetables, carrots, beans, tomatoes, fruits (especially citrus fruits), nuts and provides carbohydrates, minerals, Vitamins C and A.

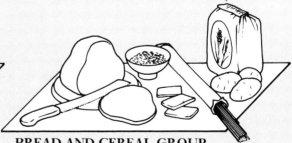

BREAD AND CEREAL GROUP
Includes bread, potatoes, rice, pasta, breakfast cereal, savoury biscuits, seeds and provides protein, carbohydrates, minerals and Vitamin B.

ENJOYING YOUR FOOD

There are three important ingredients in cooking that no money in the world can buy – imagination, flair and love. Add these to any meal and it becomes something special and memorable.

The way in which you approach the foods you are going to cook will be passed on to those you are cooking for. In theory it may seem impossible, if you are under pressure, to produce anything out of the ordinary – but applying imagination to your cooking need not take any extra time and effort. All it will involve is taking a different look at the foods you are using and not being afraid to experiment with different tastes and varieties.

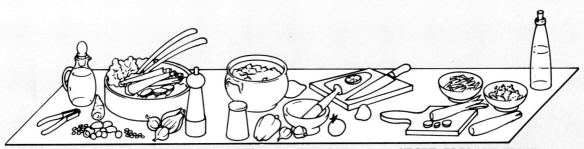

SALADS

– Stop thinking of them as a side dish – a few pieces of lettuce, a quarter of tomato, a slice or two of cucumber.

– Start experimenting with other ingredients – chopped-up spinach leaves, chunks of fennel, dried fruits, nuts, and cooked vegetables like beans are perfect ingredients.

– Change the presentation by cutting differently – for example, carrots can be grated, sliced in rings, chopped, cubed, or cut into strips.

– Break away from traditional dressings to change the flavour.

MEAT, FISH AND POULTRY

You can't change the basic ingredients but you can make them taste different simply by what you cook them with.

– A beef stew will be a revelation if you add just a few aniseed seeds or crushed cardamom seeds to it – or try orange juice.

– Add dried apricots or a spice like fenugreek to lamb dishes.

– Coat plain lamb chops with a layer of yogurt and chopped chives before serving.

– Before roasting a chicken, squeeze lemon juice over the breast and put the lemon inside the bird for an extra tangy flavour.

– With fish, concentrate as much on presentation as the actual cooking. Remember it is a colourless food so you can go to town with the garnishing – bright red strips of pepper, tomatoes, sprigs of parsley.

VEGETABLES AND FRUIT

– Always cook your vegetables in as little boiling water as possible to get the maximum flavour and nourishment – better still, you can sauté them gently in a little oil. If you cut them into small pieces they will not take so long to cook.

– For a change try eating your vegetables on their own after the main course – this way you will really be able to appreciate their flavour. A dish of freshly cooked beans, puréed spinach or carrots gently sautéed in a little oil with chopped onion and a spot of honey are all delicious on their own after a meat or fish course.

– As for fruit – start opening your eyes to a lot of possibilities in the realm of fruit drinks. Don't stop at plain orange juice – try mixing it with grapefruit or lemon.

– If you have a blender, make a delicious drink with a banana, an egg white and some good-quality bottled apple juice. Whizz for half a minute and it is ready to drink.

WHOLE HEALTH DIET

This is a diet for life – not one that you abandon after a few weeks or months. Everyone talks about a 'balanced' diet and this is what the whole health diet is. It is balanced because the foods in it are ones that provide just what your body needs.

What it does not include are the foods that many of us eat but which provide virtually nothing in the way of nutrients.

The diet is a simple one and can be divided into three sections.

FOODS YOU CAN EAT

These are the ones containing the proteins, vitamins, minerals and essential fats in good amounts, sufficient for the body to renew itself and to protect you against infection. The foods you can eat are all those from the four food groups mentioned on the preceding page.

PROTEIN-RICH FOODS
Meat, fish, eggs, cheese, milk and other milk products, peas, beans, lentils.
Note:
– eat meat, fish or eggs preferably at breakfast or lunchtime. Avoid frying these foods if you have a weight problem.
– if you already eat a lot of meat cut down on the amounts.
– when you eat cheese go for the hard varieties or cottage cheese as they are lower in fat.
– if you are overweight drink skimmed milk – no more than two glasses a day or, if you prefer, have natural yogurt.

VEGETABLES AND FRUIT
There is no variety that is not good for you. Eat them as often as you can, and certainly with every meal as they provide much of the fibre so essential in a good diet.
Note:
– aim to have at least one portion of raw vegetable each day – carrots or tomatoes are ideal.

FOODS YOU CAN EAT IN SMALL QUANTITIES

FAT
Most will be provided in your diet when you cook food or make sauces and salad dressings – it is excess of saturated fats you need to avoid. So use butter and cream sparingly and favour poly-unsaturated oils, like corn and soya.

BISCUITS AND CAKES
These add very little to your basic dietary needs. If it is hard to break the habit have them as infrequently as possible, and at times when you would normally reach for the biscuit tin go for the fruit bowl instead.

COFFEE, TEA, ALCOHOL, SOFT DRINKS
None of these beverages offers much nutritionally. Drink them by all means but don't forget there are better alternatives – fruit and vegetable juices, herbal teas.

FOODS NOT ESSENTIAL FOR HEALTH

SUGAR
Remember that it is an 'empty' calorie food. All it supplies is energy and you can get this from cereals and fruit which also have vitamins.
Sugar also needs quite a quantity of vitamins and minerals in order to be metabolised.
Note:
– all table sugars are equally bad – brown, white, raw.
– remember honey is also a sugar.

ADDITIVES, ARTIFICIAL COLOURING AND FLAVOURING
You're going to have to become a champion label reader – but it is worth it to avoid excessive intake. Most of the time your commonsense will tell you what to avoid – ice creams, cake mixes, preserved meats.

POINTS TO BEAR IN MIND
– always start the day with a good breakfast. It's an essential meal after a night without food and your body needs food right at the beginning of the day to prepare you for the mental and physical exertions that lie ahead.

– after breakfast you don't have to stick to a classic three-meals-a-day plan. If you're happier eating little and often then do so.

– if you are a little overweight the whole health diet is a pleasant way of getting rid of the extra pounds. None of the foods in it will make you put on weight – provided you don't abuse them by **over-eating**.

– to help you get started here are sample menus for two days. Given the wide variety of foods that you can eat you should find no difficulty at all in adapting yourself to a much healthier way of eating.

– cook vegetables for as short a time as possible and in very little boiling water to conserve vitamins.

– buy vegetables and fruit in season to avoid canned varieties. If you do buy canned fruit go for unsweetened varieties.

– if you are weight-watching avoid dried fruits, which have a higher sugar content.

– don't forget you can replace whole vegetables and fruit by their juice.

NUTS AND SEEDS
These are excellent mineral providers for your diet and they also contain essential fatty acids.
Note:
– if you are slimming eat seeds rather than nuts as they contain less fat.

GRAINS
Bread and cereals are an essential part of any diet as they provide the fibre the body needs to eliminate waste products.
Note:
– try to have whole grain cereals for breakfast or, if you prefer other varieties, sprinkle a couple of spoonfuls of bran or wheatgerm over them.

– refined (white) bread, flour and pasta are better than none but you'll be better off if you switch to wholemeal varieties.

– include sprouting grains in your diet – they are rich in protein and vitamins.

– remember to take enough fluids to balance the extra fibre content in your diet.

DAY ONE

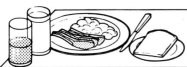

BREAKFAST
Glass of fresh, unsweetened orange juice
Scrambled egg and grilled bacon
Slice of wholemeal toast
Glass of milk

LUNCH
Glass of vegetable juice
Grilled lamb chop
Peas or fresh cabbage
Potatoes
Fresh fruit salad

DINNER
Home-made vegetable soup
Omelette with fresh herbs
Mixed salad
Natural yogurt

DAY TWO

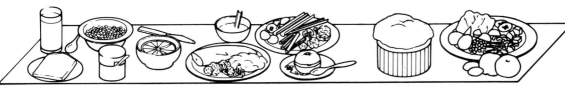

BREAKFAST
½ grapefruit
Cereal
Wholemeal toast and marmalade
Glass of milk

LUNCH
Raw vegetable platter with yogurt dip
Grilled mackerel with mustard sauce
Puréed potatoes
Spinach or broccoli
Baked apples stuffed with raisins, dates and orange rind.

DINNER
Cheese soufflé
Large mixed salad including nuts, sprouted seeds, e.g. bean shoots, or anything you fancy.
Fresh fruit

THE FIRST YEAR OF LIFE

Naturally you'll want your baby to be healthy and happy. The food he eats in his first year will lay the foundations for his future development. So, start off with the right diet and you should be well on the way to seeing a healthy child and, later on, adult.

THE FIRST SIX MONTHS

For the first months all your baby really needs is milk. And there's no doubt about it – breast milk is best of all. It contains properties that simply cannot be reproduced in commercial milks. Perhaps most important of all are the built-in protections against infection: proteins secreted by the breast which attach themselves to the lining of the baby's intestine and prevent certain infections developing. Breast milk contains living cells which can attack and destroy bacteria and viruses.

Also, the human protein in breast milk has been shown to build up resistance to many allergies such as eczema and asthma.

The Ministry of Health now recommends that babies should be breast-fed for at least four months – after that their bodies can cope with animal protein but you can continue to breast-feed for longer than this if it suits you.

BOTTLE FEED

These are a few vital points to bear in mind:
– Always make sure bottles and teats are clean and sterile.
– Never ever add extra powder to the feed – use exactly the amount suggested and always smooth the top of the scoop with a knife.
– Never add extra sugar to the feed.
– If the baby doesn't finish the bottle don't push him – just throw away the leftovers.

WHAT ELSE DOES BABY NEED?

A small baby gets thirsty too. Between feeds offer boiled water or diluted concentrated fruit juices – never give fruit squashes with artificial colourings or flavourings, or give undiluted juice on a dummy.

The only vitamin that breast milk may not provide in sufficient quantities is Vitamin D. From about four weeks you should give your baby vitamin drops which you can obtain from your local clinic – you should discuss this with your doctor first. Powdered milk contains all the essential vitamins, so you don't need to bother with extra doses until he progresses to ordinary cow's milk at about six months or later.

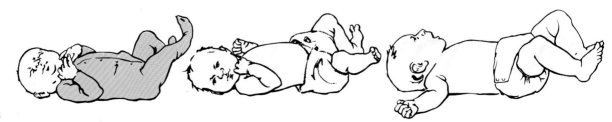

SOME FOOD SUGGESTIONS

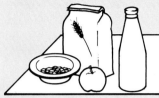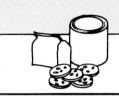

MUESLI
You don't have to use packaged baby cereals – make a baby's muesli with oat flakes and some bran or wheatgerm and soak overnight in water or fruit juice. In the morning add milk and a finely grated apple.

BISCUITS
Make healthy biscuits as a change from toast fingers. Sesame seed is ideal – use blackstrap molasses to sweeten rather than sugar or honey.

SOUP
Make your own soup – chicken or a marrow bone is ideal. Baby can have soup to start with and then the mashed vegetables from the soup as a second course – but give him his portions without salt added.

SIX MONTHS TO ONE YEAR
Don't be in too much of a hurry to introduce solid foods into baby's diet – he'll be quite happy with milk for at least the first four months but as he shows signs of being more hungry you can introduce some new tastes – on a spoon and not added to the feed.

A fat baby is not a healthy baby, so provided he is contented, sleeping well and feeding adequately there is no need to rush to stuff extra food other than milk into him.

Don't introduce a lot of different foods at once. Give baby a chance to get used to one taste before progressing to another. Unless baby is overweight you can start with a little baby rice mixed with milk – never add sugar and always offer the food half-way through a milk feed to start with.

Then you can progress to some home-made puréed broth such as chicken. Don't add salt or other seasonings. Or you can try puréed vegetables such as carrots or spinach or stewed and puréed fruit – here again no salt or sugar should be added.

Another possibility is egg yolk – but not the white, as this is hard for a small baby to digest. You can offer the egg yolk on its own or mixed with fruit or rice. After six months you can try a little grated cheese mixed in with the vegetables or minced or puréed meat. Don't give him fried or fatty foods or

leftovers – the latter will not be hygienic and the former are too difficult to digest. By eight months your baby will be able to chew, so you can offer foods with small, soft lumps.

Once the teeth come through you can give a baby a finger of toast or a piece of apple to chew on, obviously making sure you're close at hand in case he chokes. Avoid biscuits or snacks between meals – they will spoil baby's appetite and create bad habits for later on.

By the time baby is a year old he'll probably have progressed to solid foods, still in soft lumps rather than hard pieces, and be taking his drinks from a cup.

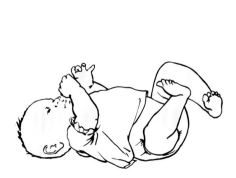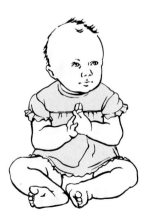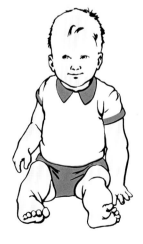

THE GROWING CHILD

Once your child has adapted to solid foods you'll
be entering perhaps the most important stage in his
life. Habits formed now can last a lifetime – so
make sure they are good ones.

Encourage your child to use his teeth – offer him
plenty of raw fruit and vegetables and, later on,
nuts. But try to avoid offering too many between-
meal snacks and be careful not to impose your own
dislikes – give your child the chance to form his
own preferences.

Your child needs foods from all the four food
groups to grow and develop, so make sure he has
balanced amounts every day. Follow the ideal diet
and adjust quantities accordingly to make sure he
has the extra amounts of calcium vital for building
bones.

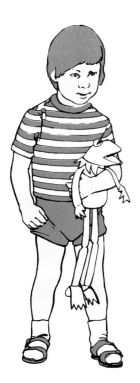

AVOID BAD EATING HABITS

At some point, usually before school age,
you are certain to come up against an
eating problem. For example, many
children suddenly turn against milk –
but there are ways round this. Make
custard, milk puddings, cheese sauces,
milk shakes with fresh fruit.

Fight like mad against falling into the
habit of offering sweets either as bribes
or rewards. Official figures show that
63 per cent of five-year-olds in England
and Wales have active tooth decay due
to too much sugar in their diet. So
sweets, biscuits and cakes, sugar on
cereals and in drinks should be avoided,
especially before your child starts school.
If he gets into the habit of not having
sweet foods he is less likely to want them
later when they are offered.

Many parents get very upset if their child
refuses to eat. Remember, if this
happens, that it is one method a child can
use to establish himself as a person in his
own right. The more fuss you make the
more he will enjoy the attention he can
arouse.

WHAT TO DO IF YOUR CHILD WON'T EAT

Keep calm – no child will starve himself
deliberately. If you are worried take him
to the doctor for a check-up and once you
are sure he is fit and healthy you can
relax. Above all avoid trying to
compensate by offering snacks between
meals. Don't let your child take over by
eating exactly what he likes. Some
children will eat nothing but meat and
no vegetables, others do it the other way
round. In either case offer the least
popular food first.

Make the food attractive when you serve
it. Cut vegetables into strips and arrange
them in patterns on the plate. Decorate
cheese on toast with strips of tomato and
sprigs of parsley, cut wholemeal bread
into different shapes – you can press
them out with animal-shaped biscuit
cutters and then toast them.

LUNCH BOX IDEAS

If your child is taking a lunch box to school make sure it's a good one. There are plenty of alternatives to a mass of sandwiches.

Try some of the following;

– A slice of quiche, fresh carrot sticks or a tomato, fresh fruit, a drink such as orange juice or apple juice.

– A boiled egg with a twist of salt, whole-meal bread and butter, pieces of lettuce and cucumber and green pepper strips, yogurt with fresh fruit.

– A ham and cheese sandwich on whole-meal bread, celery sticks, home-made biscuits made with sesame seeds.

– On a cold winter's day why not give him a small thermos of nourishing home-made soup followed by a sandwich and yogurt.

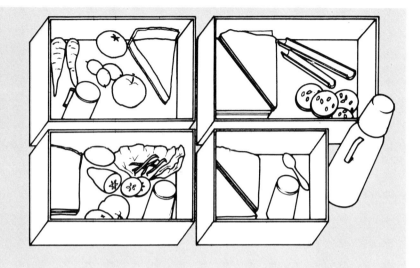

THE SCHOOL CHILD

If your child is having school dinners he may well start eating foods he previously rejected. But if when he comes home he is hungry, offer him fruit, raw vegetables or nuts and raisins to stave off the pangs until supper time.

In the evenings, after school, the young child will probably be very tired. Avoid cooking elaborate meals – something quick, tasty, nutritious and easily digested is ideal: soup, a boiled egg, welsh rarebit, cheese soufflé, a salad.

As your child gets older and has home-work to do, don't let him get into the habit of eating biscuits and cakes later in the evening. Fresh fruit or a bowl of nuts and raisins and a warm drink are much better.

Always make sure your child leaves home in the morning with a good breakfast inside him. Even if it means getting everyone up a little earlier it is well worth it – he'll work better after a good nutritious start.

A cooked breakfast of eggs, bacon or tomatoes with toast and a glass of orange juice is best of all. If he won't eat this then cereal is all right if it's muesli or any other cereal with some extra bran or wheatgerm added. In winter, porridge provides an excellent, warming start to the day.

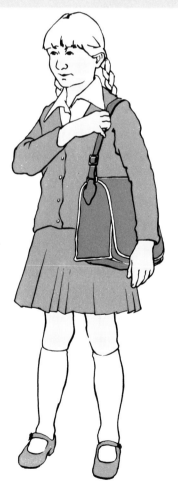

ADOLESCENCE

In adolescence a teenager is going through many physical and hormonal changes which may affect dietary needs.

Puberty, for both boys and girls, is a time when they need lots of extra energy which is best provided by plenty of good sleep and food.

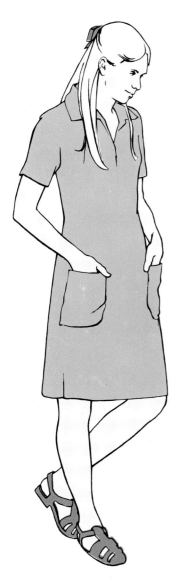

COPING WITH GROWING UP

At this time life is filling up with all kinds of pressures. There are exams to be taken, future careers to be sorted out, relationships with the opposite sex to be coped with. Altogether it can be a fairly traumatic period in many teenage lives. Above all they may not want to think as you do – and that can often mean rejecting your ideas on what they should eat as well.

Trying to force food down them 'because it's good for you' will not work now. You need to be subtle about it. Don't give up the fight altogether, because what your child eats now is just as important as it was when he was a toddler.

Try to avoid food confrontations – especially at the table. Mealtimes are the perfect opportunity for the family to get together and exchange ideas and thoughts and you can't do that if you are constantly arguing about your teenager eating all his greens.

Your best way of attack lies in being both original and subtle. Conceal wheatgerm nourishment for example in hamburgers instead of openly sprinkling it over fruit salad. Tempt your teenager to eat interesting vegetable concoctions and drink exciting fruit drinks.

Another good way to help ease any friction is to get him or her into the kitchen to cook a meal.

If you can manage it, aim to serve the evening meal early on. It will probably be the only time of the day when the whole family can be together. Serving it early gives everyone time to digest the food and also means you can be together for a while before everyone separates to do homework or go out.

Adopt a flexible attitude to meals. Try and prepare foods that can easily be stretched to include unexpected guests – that way you'll keep in touch with your teenagers' social life and make them feel their friends are always welcome.

SOME SUGGESTIONS

Since teenagers do love snacks here are five healthy snack ideas;

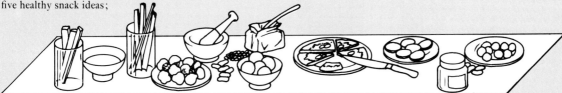

DIPS

Make up a dip with mayonnaise or yogurt. Keep it covered in the fridge together with a jug of carrots, celery sticks, cauliflower flowerets.

SEED BALLS

Make peanut or sunflower seed balls simply by crushing the nuts and mixing them with cottage cheese, curd cheese or cream cheese and rolling into walnut-sized balls.

PIZZA

Make a pizza and cut it up into biscuit-size pieces.

SWEET BISCUITS

Make delicious sweet but healthy biscuits by combining peanut butter, honey, sunflower seeds and bran in equal proportions and rolling into small balls. Keep in the fridge to be eaten when hunger strikes.

CHEESE BISCUITS

Instead of sweet biscuits make cheesy ones simply by making pastry and adding grated cheddar cheese to the mixture.

Don't stock up with junky foods like cakes and biscuits. Fill your shelves with nuts, dried fruit, seeds, home-made biscuits.

Fill your fridge with plenty of cheese, cold meats such as chicken and beef, yogurt, fresh vegetables like carrots already scrubbed and placed in a jug of water to crisp up.

The fresh fruit bowl should always be around now and not just brought out for dessert.

One of the banes of many a teenager's life is spots. A diet containing plenty of Vitamin A can be a help, so are foods rich in calcium, Vitamin D and Vitamin C.

It could be that your children become aware of healthy foods even before you do. Don't discourage them if this happens. Learn from them, let them prepare especially healthy meals for the whole family.

Be on the alert for any weight problem.

Young girls, especially, can put on extra weight as adolescents. If your child feels she is overweight then take her to the doctor to confirm this. If a diet is needed then it should be supervised by him. 'Crash' diets are a bad idea at any time, but especially during puberty. Eating less on a balanced diet will do the trick. An increasing danger at this time is that teenagers may overdo their slimming regimes. In extreme cases this may lead to psychological disturbance and the development of anorexia nervosa – where a teenager may develop very bizarre eating habits.

Be aware of what your child is doing. If he or she seems to be dieting, refusing all foods with carbohydrates, living off salads and little else, then this could be a warning sign. A talk with your doctor early on, before the situation gets out of control, is a good idea.

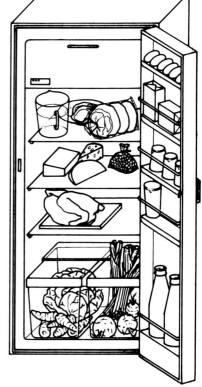

LATE TEENS AND TWENTIES

Late teens and twenties are a time of change: leaving school, starting university or college, setting off on a first job, living alone in a flat, bed-sit or digs.
Naturally parents worry whether their child will cope and if your parents have always cared about what you eat you're bound to be told 'Make sure you eat properly'.
If you've had good eating habits instilled in you from an early age you're unlikely to go completely off the rails foodwise – but it isn't easy, after years of home cooking, to have to cater for yourself.

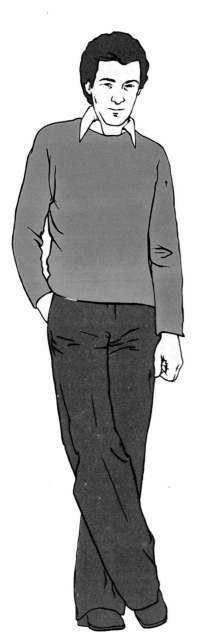

AT COLLEGE OR UNIVERSITY
For the first time perhaps you're having to handle your own finances and there are so many things that have to be paid for – lodging, books, clothes. But don't put food at the end of your list. If you eat well you'll work better and feel healthier and it need not cost a fortune.

IN HALL OR DIGS
You'll be eating college food and chances are that it will miss out on some of the things you can have in your own home if you have been following a whole health diet.
Most halls of residence have kitchens where you can prepare hot drinks and simple food. There's nothing to stop you getting salads together – there'll be space in your room to sprout your own seeds to add to it. You can also make sure you always have a bowl of fresh fruit in your room and nuts and raisins to nibble at in the evenings when you are working or chatting with friends.
At breakfast time bring your own bran to sprinkle over the cereal and a fresh orange to start the meal if it is not provided.
At lunchtime you'll probably eat in the refectory or college bar. Try not to overdo it on starchy foods. In the warmer weather it should be possible to gather together the ingredients for a simple picnic – some cheese, fruit, yogurt, ham and a hunk of wholemeal bread.
You don't have to eat puddings if they are starchy – ask for fresh fruit or yogurt instead.
Don't skip meals. There will be times when you'll be working as hard as you'll ever work – at least mentally – and you need nourishment to sustain you through hours of lectures, tutorials and revision.
When you go home for weekends stock up on basics to last through the following week. Back at college concentrate a lot on getting plenty of Vitamin C into your diet – either in fruit or from those sprouting seeds. It will give you a healthy skin and help to avoid spots breaking out.

SOME SUGGESTIONS

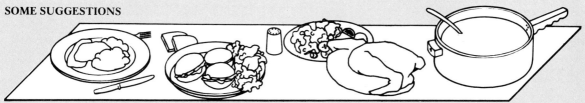

FISH
Fish for supper or lunch needn't be a grey piece of flannel in a watery liquid. Poach your white fish gently in water, with a little lemon juice or vinegar, a sliced carrot and onion. Make a cheesy sauce to go over it and top with mashed potato mixed with swede or parsnips.

HAMBURGERS
Make different hamburgers with minced beef, grated onions, an egg, chopped garlic, grated raw potatoes, chopped spinach. Grill rather than fry and serve with a green salad.

SALAD
Show your friends what a **real** salad is all about by mixing together lettuce, tomatoes, cubes of cheese, nuts, seeds, uncooked spinach leaves.
Instead of the usual oil and vinegar dressing make a yogurt dressing – natural yogurt, salt and pepper and lemon juice.

CHICKEN
If you splash out on a chicken or a joint, use the carcass or bones to make soup for the next day. Just add water to cover and some chopped carrots or leeks. Season to taste.

SOUP
You can make a meal out of soup too. A delicious vegetable soup can be made within half an hour from virtually anything you have at hand – by braising the chopped up pieces first, adding water and, if you like, a vegetable stock cube. Throw in a handful or two of brown lentils or rice and you have a nourishing meal.

IF YOU'RE LIVING ALONE
Bed-sit life can be depressing and lonely at times but whatever happens don't fall into the trap of not eating properly just because you're cooking for one.
Don't be put off by the lack of equipment in most bed-sits. It's amazing what you can achieve on just a single ring with careful timing and saucepan balancing! Keep to your old habits of having a good breakfast of fresh juice, an egg or cereal and a slice of bread. At lunchtime you'll be with the crowd, so your most important meal of the day will probably be in the evening.
Like living-in students you can sprout your own seeds for salads and you may also be able to grow herbs in pots on the windowsill.
If you are out at work you may have more time to shop each day for your evening meal.
Unless you are lucky enough to have a fridge you are going to have to come to terms with getting in fresh food each day or so and not being able to store much – but that needn't stop you from eating well.

STOCK UP A LARDER
It's worth stocking up on some foods to fall back on on those days when you've been too busy to get to the shops. Tinned sardines are an excellent standby – you can grill them on toast, make a delicious pâté or sprinkle them with lemon juice to have with a salad. Nuts and dried fruit are a must for your store cupboard and so are cereals like bran, wheatgerm, oats.
A good variety of dried herbs, such as thyme, oregano, rosemary, can change an ordinary dish into something quite special.

COOKING IS FUN
This may be the first time you've been let loose in the kitchen on your own for any length of time. Anyone who enjoys food should enjoy cooking. After a fraught day at work or lectures it is very soothing and satisfying to settle down calmly to create a meal – a few recipe books will set you off on the right track and from there you can be as creative as you like.
Experiment – that's the advantage of cooking for one.

THINK OF THE FUTURE — NOW
Prevention is better than cure, so now is the time to start adjusting your diet and get into training for a healthy middle age. Start cutting down on fatty foods now and you'll be doing your heart a favour by helping to prevent the build-up of fatty deposits and cholesterol later on. Eat less butter and opt for poly-unsaturated margarines and vegetable oils. If you take sugar in your coffee and tea, cut it out. Avoid eating too many fried foods and increase the fibre content in your diet by eating plenty of fresh fruit, vegetables, nuts and seeds; sprinkle wheatgerm and bran on dishes. Keep a close, but not obsessive, watch on your weight. Many people do less exercise after leaving school and that's when weight problems can start as muscles become flabby and fat starts to build up.

PREGNANCY

Eating for two when you're pregnant really means eating doubly well – but not in double portions. Now, more than ever before, is the time to think about those four food groups at the beginning of this chapter and make sure that you eat generously from each of them.

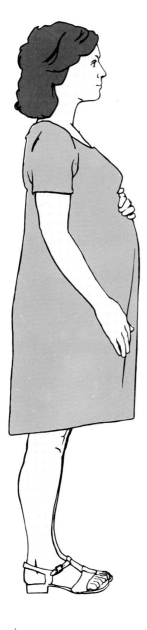

THE MILK GROUP also provides protein and calcium. During pregnancy you should have at least one pint of milk a day in some form – you don't have to drink it straight. Use it on cereals, in puddings and sauces, or take it as yogurt or an extra helping of cheese.

THE MEAT GROUP supplies protein and vitamins vital for the growth and repair of body tissues like muscles, bones, nerves, blood and teeth, and for energy. Aim to have liver or kidney at least twice a week as their iron content helps to make healthy blood, and your baby, during pregnancy, is building up an iron supply to last him for the first few months after birth.
Vitamin B in meat also ensures that muscles and nerves are in good order. If you don't eat or like meat then you should be sure to take iron supplements and include eggs in your diet.
Fish is also a good protein source. White fish is easy to digest but fatty fish like tuna, mackerel, herring, sardines have good supplies of Vitamin D – so eat a helping of these at least once a week. Canned fish with the bones included, such as sardines or salmon, are good sources of calcium, so remember to include them in your diet as well.

THE FRUIT AND VEGETABLE GROUP provides a multitude of vitamins and minerals essential for your well being and that of your baby. You should have them at least twice a day. Fruit such as oranges and other citrus fruits, and vegetables such as cabbage, broccoli and spinach are rich in Vitamin C – vital for healthy skin and blood. Have orange or grapefruit for breakfast and one of the vegetables with a main meal. Remember that cooking destroys Vitamin C, so try and have these foods raw as often as possible and if you cook them do so for as short a time and in as little water or oil as you can manage without burning.
A pregnant woman should drink at least 2 pints of liquid daily – so you can supplement the milk by drinking fruit or vegetable juices, or water.

THE BREAD AND CEREAL GROUP contains the carbohydrates for energy – and you'll need plenty of that during pregnancy, and after. It's the one group that you can cut down on if you are gaining too much weight, but check with your doctor first. You can still eat from this group in moderation. Go for foods like wholemeal bread and cereals containing bran; they provide fibre and will prevent the discomfort of constipation.
Obviously you will put on weight when you are pregnant – on average it should not be much more than 10 kilos (22 pounds). You will probably have a bigger appetite than before and want to eat more. This is fine provided you eat more of the right things.

Chapter **7**

SOME SUGGESTIONS
LIVER
You may have terrible memories of liver but it can taste delicious if cooked the right way. Here are a couple of suggestions (both are equally good for kidneys too):
Slice liver into thin strips, fry quickly in a little oil, sprinkle with lemon juice and parsley and eat at once.
Cut liver or kidneys in thin slices, again cook fast for a couple of minutes and serve with dollops of soured cream or yogurt – delicious. Eat with a green salad. Chopped liver is tasty on toast. Mash up some cooked liver, fry some finely chopped onions gently and add them to the liver. Season to taste and you have instant and nourishing pâté.

SALMON
Instead of straightforward cold tinned salmon and salad try salmon patties. Mix the salmon (and bones) with an egg and some mashed potato and a spoonful of bran or wheatgerm, season with salt, pepper and lemon juice. Make into patties, brush with a little oil and grill or bake in the oven until heated through.

A HEALTHY DRINK
If you are really under pressure at breakfast time start the day with home-made eggnog for plenty of the right nourishment. Either whisk or whizz together in the blender 2 eggs, 2 cups of milk, a few drops of vanilla flavouring and a couple of tablespoons of blackstrap molasses. You can also add any soft fruits in season.

IF YOU FEEL SICK
Many women do suffer from nausea, especially in the early stages of pregnancy. If you get morning sickness the best solution is to have a cup of tea and a piece of dry toast in bed before you get up. Then you will probably feel well enough to eat a proper breakfast later – a meal you should try not to skip. If you feel sick during the day avoid eating fried foods and also don't cook if it upsets you – cold meals and salads are just as good for you as a hot meal.

HEARTBURN
Indigestion is another of the problems of pregnancy – especially in the later stages when the baby is pressing against the stomach.
It will help to eat simple meals – nothing too spicy or over-seasoned, avoid fatty foods.
Try and have your main meal at lunchtime rather than in the evening. Always sit down quietly when you eat and rest for a while afterwards. Try not to dash around too much after a meal. If you find your digestive system simply can't cope with a large meal then break your meals up over the course of the day into nutritious snacks – but treat each snack as a meal by sitting down at the table and enjoying what you eat.

CRAVINGS
You may get cravings for a particular food – the four food groups provide a wide choice so with any luck you will hit on something that's good for you. If you don't, then try to keep a sense of proportion about it and remember that too much, say, ice cream, isn't going to benefit you or the baby much.

WHAT YOU SHOULD AVOID
Smoking – If you smoke during pregnancy – even in the early stages before your pregnancy is confirmed – you are putting your unborn child at risk. Babies born to smokers tend to be around 6 ounces lighter at birth. Smoking is unhealthy, unsociable and now is the time to stop – and never start again.
Alcohol – Although there is no proof that alcohol in moderation can harm a baby it is an appetite depressant, so if you drink a lot it may prevent you from eating properly. The occasional glass of wine or beer won't be harmful but keep it at that.

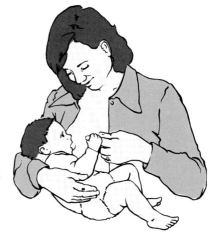

AFTER THE BABY IS BORN
If you are breast-feeding you'll need to be just as aware of your diet as during pregnancy. There will be extra demands on your calcium supply from the baby but you can balance this by eating plenty of milk, cheese and yogurt.
You can also sprinkle bone meal on your food and you should, of course, drink plenty of milk or milk products.
You'll need all the energy you can get with a new baby around – whether you are feeding him yourself or not. Brewer's yeast contains most B vitamins and is an excellent way of ensuring that the nervous system is kept healthy to help you cope with broken nights and busy days. Take it either in tablet form or sprinkled on soups, vegetable juices, etc.

MIDDLE AGE

'Life begins at forty', so the song goes, and it can for you – but you need to have the right attitudes. For many people their forties especially are the years when they start to put on weight – although the problem can start earlier. If you're a wife you're likely to have reached a threshold of boredom after fifteen or so years of cooking family meals. Now is the time to take a fresh look at cooking – remember that it is one of the most creative things you can do. So don't stick to your tried and true recipes – attempt something new at least once or twice a week to liven up those jaded taste buds. If you have teenage children now is the time to let them loose in the kitchen to cook for the rest of the family.

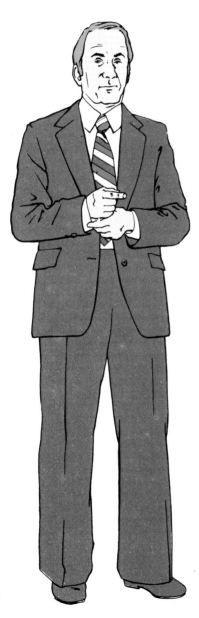

BEWARE OF HEART ATTACKS

Sadly, now is also the time when you are more likely to suffer heart attacks and even if you haven't yet had any warnings from your doctor you can do yourself (and those who love you) a favour by starting to adjust your diet to lessen the dangers now and later.

Medical research has shown that people who suffer heart attacks tend to have high levels of fat in their bloodstream – particularly cholesterol. If this level can be lowered, the risk of an attack is less. Add to a high fat level something like obesity, which affects circulation as well, and heavy smoking, and you are well on the road to disaster.

– If you haven't done so already you must stop smoking now. If you are overweight you must reduce (see Chapter 8 for suggested diets).

– To help reduce the fat levels in your system you need to know which foods to avoid in future.

Here they are:

– Top of the list in cholesterol levels are egg yolk and brains – don't have egg to eat more than three times a week – although you can use the whites as they contain no fat or cholesterol.

– Shellfish, haddock, fish roes, sardines, butter and double cream are also rich in cholesterol.

– All meat and poultry contain moderate amounts of cholesterol, so they should be eaten less frequently than before.

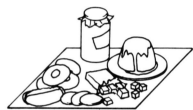

OTHER FOODS TO BE WARY OF

Anything containing extra sugar – cakes, pastries, jam, chocolate, puddings, biscuits. Eat these very occasionally if you can't do without them. If you're still taking sugar on cereals and in drinks, stop now.

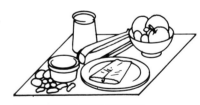

WHAT YOU CAN ENJOY

All varieties of fruit and vegetables – except avocado pears.
Cottage cheese, yogurt.
Salmon, tuna, herrings.
Nuts.
Oils made from polyunsaturated fats like corn, sunflower, soya or safflower.
Margarines and oils high in poly-unsaturates.

SOME SUGGESTIONS

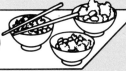

FOR A DIET INCLUDING MEAT

On a summer's day try a salad niçoise made with flaked tuna fish, tomato wedges, lettuce and strips of green and red peppers. You should also include black olives but they can be omitted on your low-fat diet.

When preparing meat be careful to trim off all excess fat and avoid frying it – grill or roast instead. Kebabs are an excellent way of serving meat with the minimum of fat – use lean lamb, marinated in lemon juice and yogurt, and brush with a very little oil before grilling. Serve with a fresh green salad and boiled rice.

Instead of buying fish fillets go for fish steaks – these too can be grilled after brushing with oil and lemon juice. A sprig of fennel on top does wonders for the flavour.

Stuffed vegetables provide a change from serving them separately.

Try green peppers – rich in Vitamin C – stuffed with lean mince and rice, or with tuna fish and chopped onion, and baked in the oven for about half an hour.

NO-MEAT MEAL IDEAS

Since vitamins are destroyed in cooking vegetables you must be sure to eat them raw as often as possible – at least once or twice a day.

Vegetables such as tomatoes, green or red peppers stuffed with cottage cheese are delicious for lunch and they look attractive too. Chop onion, chives or herbs into the cheese for extra flavour.

Take a leaf out of Chinese cookery methods – many vegetables can be cooked very fast indeed if thinly sliced and quick-fried in a little oil.

Try quick-frying slices of cabbage with a little onion and in the last couple of minutes pour over some sweet and sour sauce – delicious with rice.

If you like curry then an all-vegetable one makes a good change – you can use all kinds of combination but one based on leeks, cauliflower, a few potatoes and tomatoes and maybe some red kidney beans is ideal. Serve with rice and a green salad.

THE SECRET – make your diet interesting

Even though you'll be cutting out many foods you have relied on in the past it doesn't mean living off rabbit food for the rest of your life.

You can still start the day with a good breakfast of fruit juice or fresh grapefruit (without sugar), followed by cereal or an egg from your weekly allowance. If you are overweight don't fry the egg – have it poached or boiled instead.

You can vary breakfast by choosing some grilled lean bacon with tomatoes or grilled kipper or smoked haddock instead of the egg.

If you don't already do so, it's an excellent idea to make your own yogurt; it's a good breakfast dish when mixed with fresh fruit, nuts and cereal like oats or wheat, is low in fat and can be used in many other ways.

All you do is heat up 1 pint of skimmed milk until you can just bear to put your finger in. Add it to 1 tablespoon of commercial low-fat natural yogurt, pour it into a dish with a cover and keep in a warm place for about eight hours. To make up a new batch repeat the procedure, using a tablespoon of your own yogurt as the starter.

It may not be possible to eat your main meal at midday – it's better for your digestion if you do, but if not then try to make the evening meal easily digested by avoiding 'heavy' foods such as steak or cheese.

THINK ABOUT A MEATLESS DIET

A vegetarian diet may appeal in middle age because it is one way of cutting down on foods like fatty meats and fish, which are high in saturated fats.

A sound vegetarian diet is low in calories and you will certainly not lose out nutritionally – although you will have to plan your diet with care and use a wide selection of foods.

You can get an ample protein supply by eating cereals, legumes, peas, beans and nuts. If you include dairy products these will supply you with calcium.

But you must remember that the protein supplied by vegetables is not complete – it always needs to be complemented. So, although nuts, for instance, contain protein there is usually an amino acid missing – you must provide the missing amino acid at the same meal to obtain a protein that can be used by the body for tissue building.

So the best way round the problem – especially if you don't want to spend your day working out which food has which amino acid missing and so on – is to make sure that, if you eat nuts, seeds or grains, they are always accompanied by raw, green leafy vegetables.

Another good rule to follow is to make sure that you eat from all parts of the foods in the plant world – leaves, tubers, roots, seeds, fruits.

Remember too that eggs provide complete protein, so it makes sense to include them in your diet.

If you're thinking of taking the plunge into vegetarianism just think of all the famous, healthy and long-lived vegetarians like Bernard Shaw -- that should encourage you!

OLD AGE

As you reach retirement age you need far fewer calories in your diet but you need to be more conscious than ever of the nutrients in your food. Despite our relative wealth in the West, malnutrition and dietary deficiency are occurring more and more among the elderly.

The trouble is that, as you get older, it's easy to give in to old age – to fail to see any real purpose in life and lose interest in a lot of things, including food.

If you've just retired this is not the time to regret your old job. It is the time to do all those things you never seemed to have time for before and you'll do them so much better if you keep your body and mind healthy.

Once again the exercise you take and the food you eat will do wonders, so make good use of that extra time. Keep up with that regular exercise and take a sharp, fresh look at your diet.

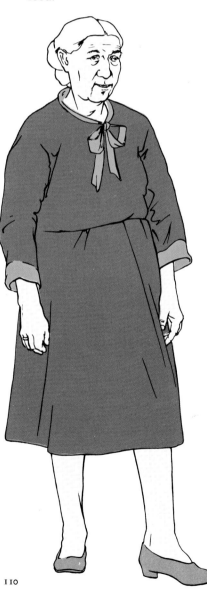

WHAT YOU NEED MORE OF NOW

PROTEIN
This is the best source of energy for you – although the body needs less of it for building cells. Since your calorie needs are lower and you are burning-up less it is better to get the calories you need from foods, high in protein, and other nutrients.

VITAMINS
You need to keep a close eye on your vitamin intake. Many elderly people suffer Vitamin D deficiencies simply because they don't get out enough – it's amazing how much sunlight can contribute. So if you are housebound you must make up for this by eating plenty of Vitamin D-rich foods such as herrings and kippers, sardines, eggs and margarine (to which Vitamin D has been added).

Vitamin C is another essential. It keeps the membranes moist and helps guard against infection. Remember that Vitamin C is not stored by the body, so you need a fresh intake each day to keep the levels right.

Eat plenty of citrus fruits each day, plus vegetables like green peppers, brussels sprouts, cauliflower – cooking these as little as possible and preferably eating them raw – as Vitamin C is easily lost in cooking water.

MINERALS
Make sure you have plenty of iron, and bear in mind that your body absorbs iron from some foods better than from others. Meat and eggs are the best sources for you.

FIBRE
One of the trials of old age – as with pregnancy – is constipation. You can make sure you are not a sufferer by including plenty of fibre in your diet rather than by taking laxatives.

Sprinkle bran over your breakfast cereal each morning – about 2 dessertspoonfuls is sufficient – or mix it into soups or stews. Eat plenty of fibre-rich foods such as raw fruit and vegetables and prefer wholemeal bread and pasta to the white varieties.

WHAT YOU STILL NEED TO AVOID
High-cholesterol foods mentioned in the previous section.

SOME SUGGESTIONS
COOKING FOR TWO

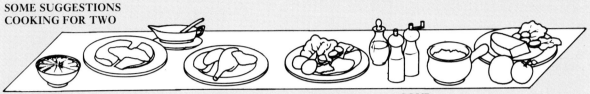

BREAKFAST
Breakfast can now be the leisurely meal you've always dreamed about. Instead of the usual foods try smoked haddock or grilled grapefruit occasionally.

CHICKEN
Make home-made mayonnaise to enjoy with cold chicken – either in pieces or chopped in. (This is equally good over cold white fish.)

JOINT OF MEAT
A joint of meat for two – just for one meal – is a waste of money. Always buy a bigger joint and then use your imagination with the leftovers.
Cold beef tastes delicious chopped up into pieces and served as a salad with a special dressing of chopped parsley, very finely chopped onions and capers mixed with a few drops of vinegar and some oil. Add salt and pepper to taste.

SOUP
If you're alone cheer yourself up on gloomy winter days with a nourishing soup made with vegetables and beans such as haricot, black or blackeye beans. Have this with a hunk of bread and a fresh salad followed by fruit.

IF THERE'S TWO OF YOU – don't be alone in the kitchen!
If you're a married woman and your husband has retired now is the time to lure him into the kitchen and share the cooking between you. Even if your husband has barely boiled an egg over the years there's nothing to stop him now from becoming an original cook. With both of you at home all day there will be three meals to prepare, so you'll be happier doing it together.
If you've never before found time to make your own bread now is the time to start.
Bread making is such a satisfying process from start to finish. The kneading is excellent exercise – and it gets rid of aggressions, if you have any! And there's that wonderful smell of freshly baked bread afterwards.

MAKE EACH MEAL SPECIAL
Retirement can be like a second honeymoon. Just the two of you, eating quietly and calmly together, no children crying or interrupting.
By experimenting with new dishes and using the extra time you have to make them attractive – and that includes laying the table properly too – you can really enjoy your food.

IF YOU'RE ALONE – AND HOUSEBOUND
Take full advantage of what is on offer from social services and voluntary organisations – like Meals on Wheels. You probably have a relative or friend who can help too by doing the shopping. Just because you can't go out and buy the food yourself don't let it make you lose interest. Many cooks get as much pleasure from planning a meal – poring over recipe books, making out a shopping list – as from the actual shopping and preparation.
If you are dependent on meals brought to you, or if you are in a home, try to make sure you are also supplied with plenty of fresh fruit, nuts and vegetables.

YOU CAN EAT WELL AND CHEAPLY
Money of course is often a problem after retirement – but that doesn't mean you have to live off bread and jam. For the few pounds you would spend on one joint of meat you can buy enough vegetables to last the week **and** keep you healthy. So although you may have to say goodbye to meat every day that doesn't mean having a poor diet.

DON'T MISS MEALS IF YOU ARE ALONE
If you are on your own it is even more tempting to skip meals now than when you were younger. Then your body could probably just cope with the punishment, but now you can't afford not to eat well.
Make it a firm rule to cook one main meal a day. Think of the advantages of being alone for meals. You can eat what you like, when you like. If you fancy having lunch at 11.30 a.m. or 2.30 p.m. you can – or supper at 4.00 in the afternoon if that's what appeals.
You can make wild experiments with cooking and you'll often be pleasantly surprised at the results.
You are bound to have friends in a similar situation to yourself. Invite them round and then go to their place.

WHY DIET?

If you're the right weight for your size you feel pretty good. You have energy, vitality. Mealtimes are a pleasure, cooking is a joy.

But if you are overweight everything changes. You may feel lethargic, sleep badly and when it comes to food there is a never-ending conflict within you about what you **should** eat and what you in fact **do** eat.

Overweight people are generally those who eat more than they personally require – and the habit can often be traced back over years.

The amount of energy you need is measured in calories or joules. The amount an individual needs to keep the body running and to use in physical exercise varies from person to person. What is certain is that as the body gets older its energy needs decrease as it works more efficiently – so if you eat the same amount of food in middle age as you did as a teenager you are almost bound to put on weight.

It takes time to become overweight – it's not simply an overnight disaster. For most people the trouble often starts when they first go out to work. It means a change of lifestyle – less exercise, lunches of

BODY TYPES

When you check your weight on a height and weight chart do bear in mind that no two people are built in the same way. Use the chart only as a rough guideline. Some research carried out in 1940 by Dr William Sheldon narrowed the field a little by putting people into three main categories.

1 Endomorphs They have small bones and muscles, large stomachs and generally soft bodies. In personality they tended to be even-tempered. They enjoyed food, creature comforts and relaxing. They also reacted slowly.

2 Mesomorphs They have big muscles and bones and spare, resistant builds. They were vigorous, aggressive types who liked to dominate.

3 Ectomorphs They have small muscles and large heads and are usually thin. In character they were inhibited, self-conscious and solitary.

Of course no-one can make hard and fast rules on personality and build. There are calm thin people and nervy fat ones. But when you check out your weight you can make allowances for your build.

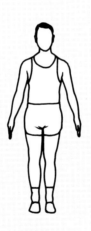
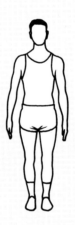
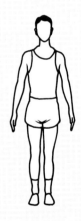
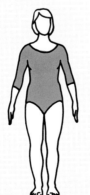
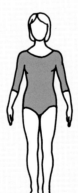
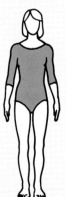

sandwiches, and snacks. The body, unwilling to waste anything, stores any excess as fat.
Once you start eating more than you need in energy terms you upset the delicate metabolic balance. To put this right takes time and that's why 'crash' diets – although they are useful – are temporary solutions and can be positively dangerous. Yes, you'll lose weight but you run two risks. First, the 'crash' diet may not provide your body with all the essential nutrients. Secondly, people who lose weight fast don't give their muscles a chance to get back into trim and may end up with a lot of unattractive flab.

What you should aim for when you diet is a change in eating habits. In this chapter we look at three different 'crash' diets. Most people like an incentive to get them on the right path. But none of these diets should be followed for any length of time. After that your aim should be to stick to a good, balanced diet like the one in Chapter 7 – cutting down on amounts to suit your needs. In the long run this will get rid of those extra pounds and you'll never see them again.

HEIGHT AND WEIGHT CHART
This chart provides just a guideline for you to use as a starting point. By checking off what your weight should be it gives you something to aim for.

Height without shoes ft in	Small frame st lb st lb	Medium frame st lb st lb	Large frame st lb st lb
MEN			
5 1	8 0 – 8 8	8 6 – 9 3	9 0 – 10 1
5 2	8 3 – 8 12	8 9 – 9 7	9 3 – 10 4
5 3	8 6 – 9 0	8 12 – 9 10	9 6 – 10 8
5 4	8 9 – 9 3	9 1 – 9 13	9 9 – 10 12
5 5	8 12 – 9 7	9 4 – 10 3	9 12 – 11 2
5 6	9 2 – 9 11	9 8 – 10 7	10 2 – 11 7
5 7	9 6 – 10 1	9 12 – 10 12	10 7 – 11 12
5 8	9 10 – 10 5	10 2 – 11 2	10 11 – 12 2
5 9	10 0 – 10 10	10 6 – 11 6	11 1 – 12 6
5 10	10 4 – 11 0	10 10 – 11 11	11 5 – 12 11
5 11	10 8 – 11 4	11 0 – 12 2	11 10 – 13 2
6 0	10 12 – 11 8	11 4 – 12 7	12 0 – 13 7
6 1	11 2 – 11 13	11 8 – 12 12	12 5 – 13 12
6 2	11 6 – 12 3	11 13 – 13 3	12 10 – 14 3
6 3	11 10 – 12 7	12 4 – 13 8	13 0 – 14 8
WOMEN			
4 8	6 8 – 7 0	6 12 – 7 9	7 6 – 8 7
4 9	6 10 – 7 3	7 0 – 7 12	7 8 – 8 10
4 10	6 12 – 7 6	7 3 – 8 1	7 11 – 8 13
4 11	7 1 – 7 9	7 6 – 8 4	8 0 – 9 2
5 0	7 4 – 7 12	7 9 – 8 7	8 3 – 9 5
5 1	7 7 – 8 1	7 12 – 8 10	8 6 – 9 8
5 2	7 10 – 8 4	8 1 – 9 0	8 9 – 9 12
5 3	7 13 – 8 7	8 4 – 9 4	8 13 – 10 2
5 4	8 2 – 8 11	8 8 – 9 9	9 3 – 10 6
5 5	8 6 – 9 1	8 12 – 9 13	9 7 – 10 10
5 6	8 10 – 9 5	9 2 – 10 3	9 11 – 11 0
5 7	9 0 – 9 9	9 6 – 10 7	10 1 – 11 4
5 8	9 4 – 10 0	9 10 – 10 11	10 5 – 11 9
5 9	9 8 – 10 4	10 0 – 11 1	10 9 – 12 0
5 10	9 12 – 10 8	10 4 – 11 5	10 13 – 12 5

SIX WAYS TO DIET SUCCESSFULLY

If you are overweight because you're eating too much, it is a form of addiction. You know you should stop but you keep putting off the evil moment. Or maybe you occasionally try to lose weight – especially in the summertime with the incentive of summer holidays and sun-bathing –

only to go back to square one within a few weeks or months.

Like any addiction, overeating is a hard habit to break – but it **can** be done. Before and during your dieting follow this six-point plan.

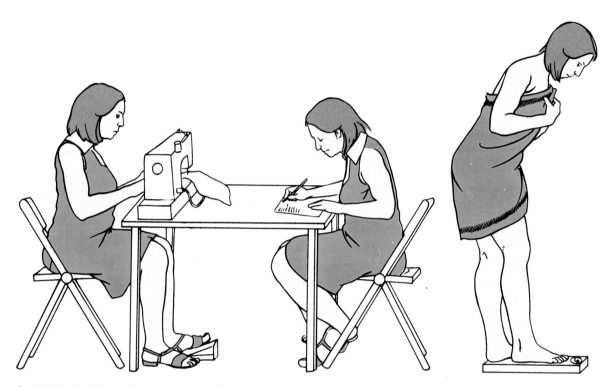

1 MOTIVATE YOURSELF

Think positive thoughts, every day, about how much happier and healthier you will be when you've lost that extra weight.

You are far less likely to run the risk of suffering from a multitude of major and minor illnesses like heart disease, bronchitis, arthritis, back pain, flat feet, diabetes, infections, shortness of breath and tiredness.

You may find that your guilt about being overweight has made you unsociable and lonely. Combat this by joining a day or evening class and developing new interests.

If you don't know how to sew, for instance, now's the time to learn – then you'll be able to take in all your clothes yourself!

2 MAKE A LIST

Give yourself a bit of a jolt by listing, honestly, what you eat now. Check this list off against the balanced diet in Chapter 7 and see how many foods you are eating from the non-essential or small-amount categories.

3 SET A TARGET

You'll see from the height and weight charts what you should weigh or you may know, from distant memories, your ideal weight. Aim to achieve this in a reasonable length of time – not too soon, which would be discouraging if you didn't meet the target. If you have a lot to lose set a target to lose some of it and then set a new target when you've achieved the first stage.

Use any notable date in your diary as a target date – a holiday, your next birthday, your wedding anniversary. Ring the day round in red – this is your D day and don't forget it!

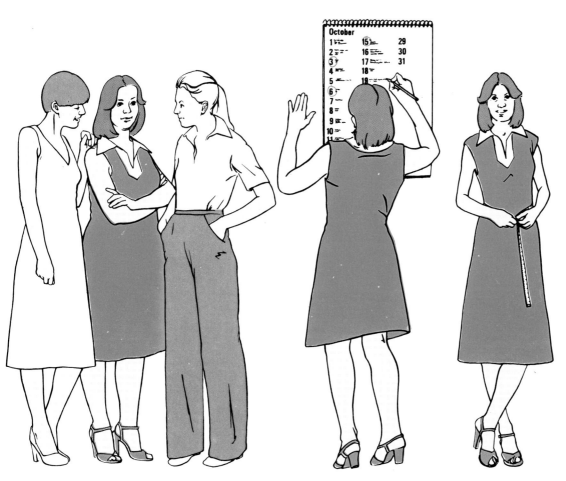

4 FRIENDS CAN HELP

Get everyone you can on your side to help fight the battle of the bulge. Seek out the healthy eaters – they can put you on the right path.

But don't rely on your friends to keep an eye on you in case you transgress. You must make yourself your sternest judge and rely on your own conscience to nag you if you sneak a forbidden bar of chocolate or a cream bun.

5 KEEP A RECORD

Once you start your new way of eating, keep a periodic record of your intake, say, after the first month, to compare with your first list. Ring round in red any foods you shouldn't have eaten, like sugar or solid fats. This record will probably cheer you up immensely as you realise what a vast improvement your new eating habits are showing.

6 REMEMBER

When you make that decision to lose weight it is going to be a lifelong one with no going back. What you are doing is changing your eating pattern. As you approach your ideal weight you may allow yourself some of your old favourites, but in moderation, although you'll probably be surprised to find your cravings, say, for sweet things, have vanished. Most people, for instance, who give up sugar in tea or coffee, can't bear to return to it.

Your new way of eating may be uncomfortable to start with but in the end you'll wonder why you didn't take the step years ago and what all the fuss was about.

RAW FOOD DIET

This is a diet you should try once in a while, whether you are overweight or not, because it seems to eliminate toxins from the body and leaves you feeling revitalised.

It should really be called the 'Makes You Feel Good' diet because that's just what it will do. A couple of days – three at the most – on this diet will leave you feeling refreshed. Your skin will be clearer and instead of just feeling well, you'll probably feel positively healthy.

The diet consists simply of raw fruits and vegetables. In this way you're going to get the maximum number of vitamins – since some are destroyed when these foods are cooked. You will also get an excellent amount of fibre into your system to stimulate it to work more efficiently at processing the food.

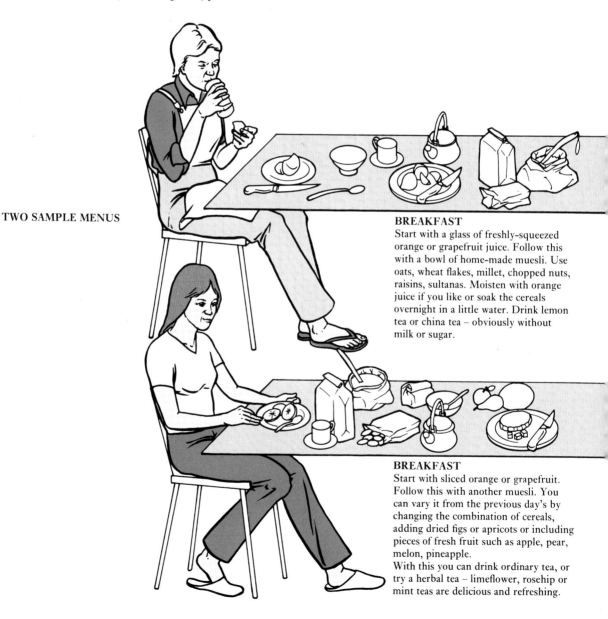

TWO SAMPLE MENUS

BREAKFAST
Start with a glass of freshly-squeezed orange or grapefruit juice. Follow this with a bowl of home-made muesli. Use oats, wheat flakes, millet, chopped nuts, raisins, sultanas. Moisten with orange juice if you like or soak the cereals overnight in a little water. Drink lemon tea or china tea – obviously without milk or sugar.

BREAKFAST
Start with sliced orange or grapefruit. Follow this with another muesli. You can vary it from the previous day's by changing the combination of cereals, adding dried figs or apricots or including pieces of fresh fruit such as apple, pear, melon, pineapple.
With this you can drink ordinary tea, or try a herbal tea – limeflower, rosehip or mint teas are delicious and refreshing.

WHEN TO GO ON THE DIET

Summertime is the obvious choice when there are plenty of fresh fruits and vegetables around and the weather is warm. But any time of year is right. If you go out to work then a weekend is quite a good moment for your first attempt at the diet. The foods you may not eat may look restrictive but you'll be surprised how enjoyable you'll find what you **can** eat.

HOW IT WORKS

The diet is simple. There is no calorie counting or weighing involved. All you have to do is choose whatever you want to eat from a vast variety of raw fruits and vegetables.

WHAT YOU CAN EAT

Any variety of vegetable – raw and chopped, sliced, grated or pulped. Any kind of raw fruit or fresh fruit juice. Nuts – fresh and uncooked. Seeds – sesame, sunflower, pumpkin. Dried fruits – figs, raisins, dates, apricots, prunes, etc.

WHAT YOU MUST NOT EAT

No cooked food of any kind whatsoever. No meat, poultry, fish. No dairy foods such as milk, cheese, cream, yogurt. No eggs. No alcohol or soft drinks. If possible avoid tea and coffee too. If you smoke you probably won't feel in the mood for it – especially if you cut out tea, coffee and alcohol. In fact if you want to give it up, this is a good time.

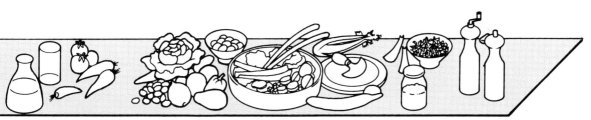

LUNCH AND DINNER

Start with a glass of tomato juice or, if you prefer, more orange juice. Mix together a salad of lettuce, thin sliced red or white cabbage, some tomatoes, pieces of fennel, cucumber, thinly sliced onion, red or green pepper. Make the salad as big or small as you like and sprinkle it generously with chopped nuts and seeds such as sesame or sunflower. For dessert have a plate of fresh or dried fruits – or a combination of the two. In winter satsumas and dried figs go perfectly. In summer try fresh pears and dried apricots. Drink mineral water with lunch. In the evening have a soothing camomile tea.

BETWEEN-MEAL SNACKS

During the day you may feel peckish. It's easy to keep within the diet and avoid the coffee and biscuits you might normally reach for. In the morning prepare carrot and celery sticks and put them in a jug of water in the fridge to crisp up. Nibble on them whenever you like, or have a handful of nuts and raisins.

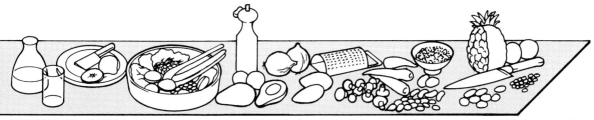

LUNCH AND DINNER

Start with a glass of raw vegetable juice. Vary the salad from the day before by making it up with slightly different ingredients. Try slices of chicory, grated carrot, chunks of celery, raw mushrooms and pieces of ripe avocado pear, sprinkled with lemon juice – you can afford to splash out on this diet. You can also include fresh orange or grapefruit or pineapple. Sprinkle the whole salad either with nuts or with sprouted grains like mung beans, alfalfa or fenugreek (for an unusual curry flavour). For dessert you can make another salad – with fruit this time. Use only fresh or dried fruits – nothing tinned. Finish the meal with a cup of herbal tea or ordinary tea.

This diet can act as an ideal introduction to a full slimming diet. It will help you to get used to doing without all those things you think you crave – sugar, cream and so on. You won't find it hard to follow this diet even if you have to eat out. Most restaurants can provide a salad – and the kind they provide is a good test of how enterprising the place is!

LOW CARBOHYDRATE PLUS

The trouble with so many diets – the faddy kinds that use only one or two foods – is that they are so hard to stick to. You get so bored with eating just bananas or cottage cheese – and it's not good for your body either to deprive it for any length of time of several essential nutrients not contained in these foods.

Low carbohydrate/high protein diets have always been popular because they are not so limited. You eat approximately normal foods but cut out the really starchy kinds and the foods that have a high sugar content. Because you are eating less it will also help you to establish your new eating pattern – one that you'll be able to stick with.

This is an easy diet to keep up away from home too. If you have to eat out in restaurants you can easily adapt your meal there to your diet.

The diet limits you to between 1200 and 1500 calories a day. The average woman needs around 2000 calories and a man around 2800 – so you can see that your calorie intake is considerably reduced and you will lose weight.

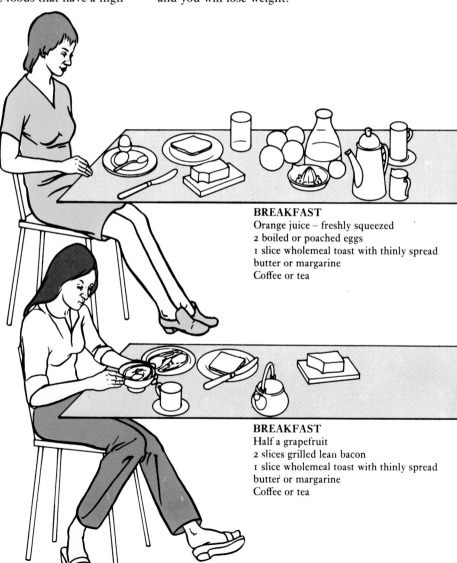

TWO SAMPLE MENUS

BREAKFAST
Orange juice – freshly squeezed
2 boiled or poached eggs
1 slice wholemeal toast with thinly spread butter or margarine
Coffee or tea

BREAKFAST
Half a grapefruit
2 slices grilled lean bacon
1 slice wholemeal toast with thinly spread butter or margarine
Coffee or tea

PROTEIN DIET

HOW THE DIET WORKS

You should not follow this diet for longer than four weeks at a time. After this you can revert to the wholehealth diet so that you are getting a completely balanced intake of foods, but by then you should not be feeling so strongly the urge to eat large quantities and will probably continue to lose weight.

To get you started here's a menu for one day of the diet. You can vary your breakfast by having cereal (without sugar of course) instead of eggs. The other meals can be changed by substituting different meats – beef, lamb etc. – but they should always be grilled or roasted. A 4 oz portion of meat or fish is ample and to go with it you should avoid potatoes and have instead vegetables like broccoli, green beans, or tomatoes.

You should also not take any extra sugar with your food – cut it out of tea and coffee and don't sprinkle it on your cereal.

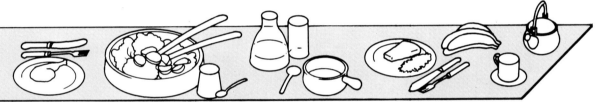

LUNCH
Grilled chicken leg
Small lettuce, tomato and apple salad –
no dressing
Natural yogurt

DINNER
Glass of any vegetable juice or bowl of clear soup
4 oz fillet of white fish – poached or grilled
Portion of spinach
1 small banana
Coffee or tea

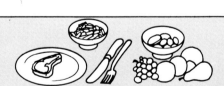

LUNCH
Grilled lamb chop
1 cupful green beans
Small fruit salad

DINNER
Bowl of clear vegetable soup
4 oz cod steak – grilled or poached
Portion of broccoli or a small salad
1 apple or pear
Coffee or tea

NIBBLE & SNACK DIET

This is an ideal weight-reducing diet for anyone who can't bear the thought of eating less just three times a day.

Many fat people have got that way by eating between meals. The difference in this diet is that you're not going to be having snacks between main meals. Each snack is a meal in itself and you are allowed six snack meals a day.

Anyone working at home who finds it hard to keep away from the fridge during the day will probably enjoy this sort of diet.

TWO SAMPLE MENUS

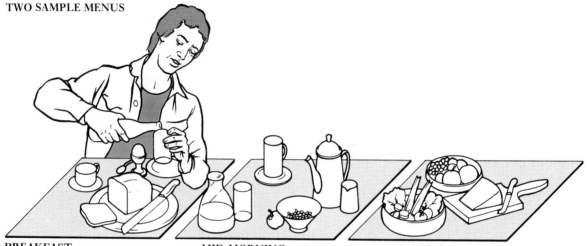

BREAKFAST
Orange juice
A boiled egg
1 slice wholemeal bread
Coffee or tea without sugar

MID-MORNING
A handful of nuts and raisins or an apple
Fresh fruit juice or vegetable juice or coffee or tea without sugar

LUNCH
Cheese salad – cheddar or cottage cheese with lettuce, tomato, cucumber
Fresh fruit

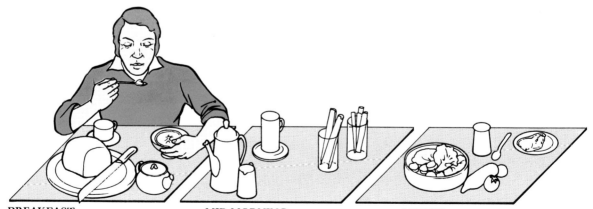

BREAKFAST
Half a grapefruit
A poached egg
1 slice wholemeal bread
Coffee or tea without sugar

MID MORNING
Carrot or celery sticks
Coffee or tea without sugar

LUNCH
Salad of lettuce, tomato, cucumber with a slice of ham
Natural yogurt

HOW IT WORKS

You eat when you feel hungry but you should only eat enough to take the edge off your appetite. Your ideal calorie count per day should not exceed the 1200 mark. If you do exceed it then you must cut down the next day.

You can eat more or less what you want but you must cut out all foods high in sugar, such as cakes and biscuits, and avoid bread, butter and jam meals.

A DAY'S MENU

Below are two examples of one day's suggested eating. You can vary it as you wish, making sure you keep within the calorie limit.

REMEMBER

If you choose to go on this diet you **must not cheat.** For the diet to work and for you to lose weight *all* your six meals each day must be snack meals. You won't lose a single pound if you have main meals and snacks in between as well!

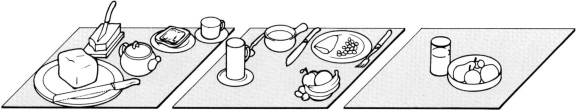

MID AFTERNOON
Slice of ham on wholemeal bread with thin spread of butter or margarine
Coffee or tea without sugar

DINNER
Small bowl of clear soup
4 oz lean meat, chicken or fish
Cup of green beans – no gravy
Fresh fruit
Coffee or tea

BEFORE BED
Cup of milk – hot or cold
An apple or a pear

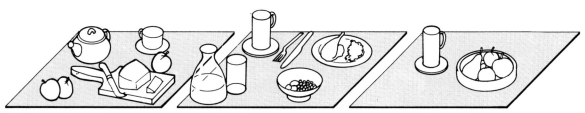

MID AFTERNOON
Chunk of cheese and a sliced apple
Coffee or tea without sugar

DINNER
Vegetable juice
4 oz lean meat, chicken or fish
Portion of spinach
Small portion of dried fruit
Coffee or tea

BEFORE BED
Cup of milk – hot or cold
An apple or a pear

RELAX-IN A HOME THAT'S SAFE

Twenty people die each day from accidents in the home and many more thousands are injured, so it makes sense to check that your home is as safe as it can be – you'll feel more relaxed too, especially if you have young children.

The Kitchen is potentially the most dangerous place in the house – the majority of accidents occur here: burns, scalds, falls, suffocation from plastic bags or fire. Check the following points to reduce the risks:

THE KITCHEN

1 Keep all matches and any flammable fluids out of reach of children.

2 Use flame-resistant fabrics for curtains, blinds.

3 Never leave fires, ovens, hot plates, gas rings unattended or unguarded if there are children about.

4 Never dry clothes near an unguarded heat source.

5 Hook up flexes of any electrical equipment so that objects like irons can't be knocked over, or the flex catch fire on a cooking area.

6 When cooking turn pan handles or kettle spouts away from front of cooker.

7 Have any gas appliances checked regularly for faults and make sure the kitchen is well ventilated.

8 If you're going away for more than twenty-four hours turn off gas and electricity at the mains.

9 Keep chemical cleaners of any kind either in a locked cupboard or well out of the reach of small children.

10 Make sure your kitchen floor has a non-slip surface. If you spill anything, wipe it up at once.

11 If you break anything like glass or china, sweep it up, don't pick up the pieces. Wrap well in lots of paper before throwing away.

12 Don't keep heavy items high up and don't stand on a chair to reach things – it's worth buying a stable pair of steps.

13 If you have children make sure they keep their toys out of your working area. Better still, make some sort of divider between their area and yours, especially while you are cooking.

14 Keep all polythene bags away from children – either throw them out at once or store in a safe place.

15 Always remove doors or lids of old cookers, fridges, freezers.

16 Have a basic first-aid kit on hand in the kitchen – just in case.

The other areas of the house should also be checked for safety.

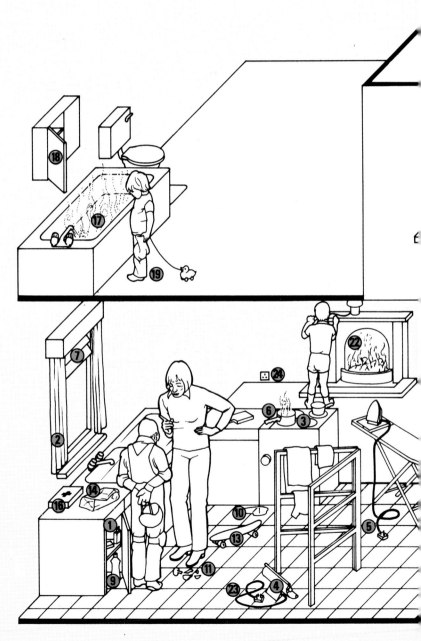

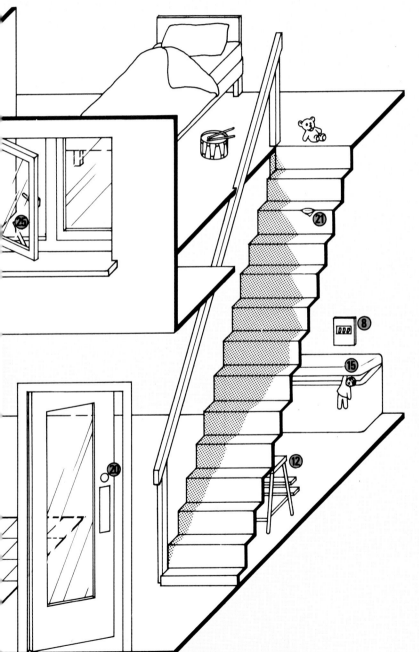

THE BATHROOM
17 Have a rubber safety mat in the bath and always run cold water in first.
18 If you have a medicine chest, make sure it is approved by the British Standards Institute. It should have a good lock. You should throw away all medicines and pills left over after a treatment.
Either flush them down the toilet or take them to your local chemist. It's a good idea to keep your medicine chest in a less accessible room than the bathroom.
19 Never leave a young child alone in the bath for **any** reason.

THE HALL
20 Have a good lock on the front door to stop children running out into the road.
21 Make sure stairs are well lit and that carpet is checked for tears, holes, firm fitting.

THE REST OF THE HOUSE
22 Always have a fireguard in front of an open gas or electric fire if there are children around.
23 Make sure plugs and equipment are properly fixed.
24 Have safety switches on all sockets or buy blind plugs to fit over open sockets.
25 Have adequate, child-proof locks on windows on the stairway and in the nursery or playroom.

CALORIE CHART

A

No. of Calories per oz

Aerated drinks	10
Ale	10
Almonds	170
Anchovies	40
Apple: fresh (4 oz)	15
baked	10
Apricot: fresh	5
dried	50
Artichoke	5
Asparagus, fresh	5
Avocado pear, without stone	25
Aubergine	5

B

Bacon: lean, fried in own fat	125
streaky fried in own fat	149
Bananas, fresh	15
Beans: baked	26
broad	12
butter	25
french	2
haricot	25
runner	2
Beef: roast	64
steak grilled	85
burger	70
Biscuits: cream cracker	125
sweet	158
digestive	137
Blackberries, raw	10
Blackcurrants, raw	10
Bloaters, grilled	75
Brazil nuts	180
Bread, 1 slice = 1 oz	70
Broccoli	5
Brussels sprouts, boiled	5
Butter	226

C

Cabbage, boiled or raw	5
Cake	85–150
Carrots, boiled or raw	6
Cauliflower, boiled	5
Celery, raw	3
Cereals:	100
All Bran	90
cornflakes	105
muesli	105
Puffed Wheat	105
Cheese: cheddar	120
cottage	30

No. of Calories per oz

Cheese: cream	230
edam	88
stilton	135
Cherries, fresh, with stones	11
Chestnuts, raw, shelled	40
Chicken, roast	55
Chocolate: milk	167
plain	155
Cider	10
Coca-Cola	12
Cocoa	128
Coconut, dessicated	170
Cod: fried	40
steamed	25
Coffee, black	0
Corn, sweet	25
Courgettes, boiled	5
Crab, boiled	35
Cranberries, raw	5
Cream: single	60
double	130
Cucumber	3
Custard, prepared	30

D

Damsons, raw, with stones	9
Dates, with stones	61
Doughnuts	100
Duck, roast	90
Dumplings	60

E

Eel, conger, fried	72
Egg: boiled	55
fried	70
scotch	75
Endive, raw	3

F

Figs: fresh	12
dried	60
Fish fingers	50
Flounder, fried	42
Flour, white or wholemeal	95

G

Gammon	60
Glucose	110
Goose, roast	90

No. of Calories per oz

Gooseberries, fresh	10
Grapes: black	14
white	17
Greengages, fresh	13
Grouse, roast	50
Guinness	10

H

Haddock: fried	50
steamed	30
Hake: fried	60
steamed	30
Hamburger, fried	70
Heart, roast	68
Herring: fried	65
baked	50
roe, fried	74
Honey	82

I

Ice cream, plain	60

J

Jams, stoned fruit	75
Jelly	23

K

Kale, boiled	10
Kidney: fried	57
braised	30
Kippers, grilled	31

L

Lager	10
Lamb chop: grilled	75
roast	74
Lard	260
Leeks, boiled	7
Lemon	4
Lemonade	6
Lemon juice	2
Lemon squash	36
Lentils, boiled	25
Lettuce	3
Lime juice cordial	32
Liver, calf, fried	74
Lobster, boiled	35

Loganberries, fresh	5	Peppers, sweet	5	Spring greens, boiled	3
Luncheon meat	95	Pheasant, roast	60	Strawberries, fresh	7
		Pilchards, tinned	55	Suet	260
M		Pineapple, fresh	10	Sugar	112
		Pistachio nuts	168	Sultanas	70
Mackerel, fresh	55	Plaice: fried	40	Swedes, boiled	5
Mandarins, fresh	10	steamed	14	Sweetbreads	50
Margarine	226	Plums, raw	10	Syrup, golden	85
Marmalade	75	Pork: roast	90		
Marrow, boiled	2	Pork chop, grilled + bone	90	**T**	
Melon	5	Potatoes: boiled	25		
Milk: fresh	20	chips	70	Tangerines, fresh	10
evaporated	45	roast	35	Tapioca	100
skimmed	10	Prawns, meat	30	Tapioca pudding	37
Mulberries, raw	10	Prunes, dried	40	Tea	0
Mushrooms, fried	60	Pumpkin	4	Tomato: raw	4
Mussels, boiled	25			fried	20
		Q		Tongue, ox, cooked	85
N				Treacle, black	75
		Quinces	7	Tripe, boiled	30
Nectarines, with stones	13			Trout, steamed	40
		R		Tuna, tinned	70
O				Turbot, steamed	30
		Rabbit, stewed	50	Turkey, roast	55
Oatmeal	115	Radish	5	Turnips, boiled or raw	3
Oatmeal porridge	15	Raisins	70		
Oil, vegetable	250	Raspberries, raw	7	**V**	
Olives	30	Rhubarb, stewed without sugar	1		
Olive oil	265	Rice	35	Veal: fried	61
Onion: raw	7	Rice pudding	40	roast	66
fried	100	Ryvita	98	Venison, roast	55
Orange	10			Victoria Sandwich	134
Orange juice	11	**S**		Vinegar	0
Orange squash	39				
Oxtail	25	Sago, pudding	35	**W**	
Oysters, raw	15	Salad cream	110		
		Salami	115	Walnuts	150
P		Salmon, fresh	55	Watercress, fresh	4
		Sardines, tinned	84	Whelks, meat	25
Pancakes	85	Sausage: pork, fried	93	Whisky	65
Parsnip, raw or boiled	15	beef, fried	80	White sauce: savoury	41
Partridge, roast	60	Scallops, steamed	30	sweet	47
Pasta, plain or egg	95	Scampi, steamed	85	Whitebait, fried	150
Pastry: flaky	167	Scone	100	Whiting: steamed	25
short	157	Semolina, pudding	37	fried	55
Pâté	132	Sherry, dry	30	Wine: light	20
Peach, fresh	60	Shrimps, raw or boiled	32	heavy	40
Peanuts	170	Skate, fried	70		
Pear, fresh	10	Sole: steamed	25	**Y**	
Peas: fresh	15	fried	50		
frozen	20	Soya flour	95	Yeast, fresh	25
dried	30	Spinach	7	Yogurt: low fat	15
tinned	24	Spirits	approx. 70	fruit	30
		Sprats, fried	125		

INDEX

INDEX

Trachea, windpipe, 30–1

U

Ulcer, peptic, 10
Untidiness, tension due to, 72
Urethra, 36
Urinary system, 25, 36
Uterus, 39

V

Vagina, 39
Vegetables, 94, 95, 96
    carbohydrate content of, 47
    fat content of, 49
    during pregnancy, 106
    protein content of, 51
    raw, 120–1
Vegetarians, vegetarian diets, 51, 109
Veins, 34
Vitamins, 44–5, 52–3, 110
    A, 49, 52, 94
    B group, 53, 94, 106
        B1, 16, 44
        B12, 16, 52
    C, 52, 94
        for the old, 110
        during pregnancy, 106
    D, 26, 49, 52, 94
        for babies, 98
        for the old, 110
        during pregnancy, 106
    E, 49, 53
    K, 49, 53

W

Walking, 92, 93
Waste products, 34
    see also urinary system
Weight and height chart, 113
Windpipe, trachea, 30–1

Y

Yoga, 90–1

Z

Zinc, 55